THE LATE BLOOMER AND HER TWO POLAR BEARS

A Personal Story of Living with Bipolar Through Sexual and Domestic Violence

Jacqueline Ellwood

First published by Busybird Publishing 2022

Copyright © 2022 Jacqueline Ellwood

ISBN:
978-1-922691-35-4 (paperback)
978-1-922691-36-1 (ebook)

This book is copyright. Apart from any fair dealing for the purposes of study, research, criticism, review, or as otherwise permitted under the Copyright Act, no part may be reproduced by any process without written permission. Enquiries should be made through the publisher.

Cover image: Jacqueline Ellwood
Cover design: Busybird Publishing
Layout and typesetting: Busybird Publishing

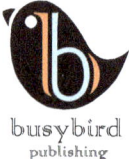

Busybird Publishing
2/118 Para Road
Montmorency, Victoria
Australia 3094
www.busybird.com.au

Extract reprinted with permission from *Too Soon Old, Too Late Smart* by Gordon Livingstone, Hachette Australia, 2005.

For more information visit: **www.twopolarbears.com.au**

To Jason, for all the strength you have always shown and the support you have always given me. It is through your example that I have learned to be stronger than I have ever been and it has, in return, shown me how to commit, which eventually made my dreams come true.

And to Susan. For all your patience while I was learning what was right in life and what I was worthy of. You're an incredible role-model so many women and I'm blessed to now call you my friend.

Author's Note

I feel the need to let you know that this is not a researched, scientific, data-based book. This is not a book that will provide a precise pathway to give you, the reader, answers to why bipolar exists nor is it a book to provide a concise path to take for you or a loved one who has been bestowed with it. My pathway through life so far would resemble a manic snail trail to get to whatever looked shiny and immediately took my fancy, in between bouts of trying to stay afloat. Graceful it was not, but colourful it has been so far.

This book is a work of my memories, made up of true stories. It is said that people who recall events have the memory of an elephant; well, I carry the whole herd within my brain and it can be bloody annoying to people who know me because they know I'm right. As bold a statement as that is, people who know me know it to be true: it's all five senses in recollection stereo.

Throughout this book, the names of all the people mentioned have been changed in order to protect their privacy, even the innocent. It was never my wish to name and shame anyone, especially members of my family, biological or marital. In saying all of that, though, it's not a matter of the truth getting in the way of a good story because, believe me, the truth is a hell of a lot funnier and better than any nonfiction I could ever think up in my crazy, cartooned mind.

I look forward to the day it becomes apparent to everyone that just because you've been diagnosed with bipolar it doesn't give someone the option to see whatever befalls you as completely your fault. Domestic or sexual violence is not something I invited into my life. My DNA being somehow defective compared to an average person's didn't make the abuse I endured a logical outcome.

I choose to no longer hold on to the anger and bitterness that I grasped onto so tightly for so long. It circulated in my mind over and over, in a mental landscape where justice never prevailed. I became self-destructive, I imploded, but then I suppose if it never happened, I would never have realised how resilient I am. It's only now I can acknowledge the pain and sit with the grief, feeling its full impact like it was yesterday, but knowing I've learned from it. Now much wiser, I am more mindful and would like other women to learn from my experiences.

All I hope is that from this book people may start to see into the life of someone they never understood. In no way am I a poster girl for this ailment – we can't be placed into a specific box. But to stand in as an example to help others understand those who have a serious mental illness and been a victim of domestic or sexual violence, I am more than willing to do.

If you are someone who has had similar experiences with abuse or sexual violence, I want you to know that there is always someone out there to listen, acknowledge what you've been through and help you on your journey to recovery. I want you to unequivocally know that you didn't ask for it.

Jackie

Contents

1968	2	2016 – November	215
1972	11	2016 – November	219
1982 – March	15	2015-2016	223
1980s	19	2017	231
1970s	23	2021	235
1982-1984	27	**Finding an Anchor in the Midst of the Storm:** Help for Women in Abusive Relationships	241
1985	36		
1985 – July	40		
1986	45		
1988	50	References	250
1989	54		
1995	61	**Appendix A** Relationship Warning Signs: Look Before You Leap!	251
1997	68		
1998	72		
2001	80	**Appendix B** Family Violence Services for Victim Survivors	254
2001 – September	84		
2002	90		
2004	97	Thank you	256
2005	107		
2006	112		
2007	116		
2008	123		
2009	128		
2010	142		
2011	152		
2012 – May	167		
2012 – July	174		
2012 – July	185		
2015 – March	188		
2015 – May	193		
2016 – September	206		

July 2020

...Then too there was your great-grandmother Mary Hobbs, on Mum's side, who was diagnosed as suffering from senile dementia and insanity. This was in 1913, when she was seventy-three, and had twice tried to 'give up life' once by (fully clothed) trying to drown herself in a bath of water and, ultimately, the event which led to her being hospitalised, by throwing herself off the platform and in front of an approaching train at Newmarket railway station.

The reason, if that is the right word: someone had been trying to murder her, there was blood everywhere and she had been 'shamed and disgraced' by the conduct of her daughters, who were bad women and running a bad house.

She had been refusing food for two days when she was examined and was confused about the day, month and year and her memory was otherwise 'very defective'

That's the best I can make of the examining doctors report on her admission to the Reception House at Kew on 31 December 1913.

Mary was seventy-three at the time and she died still in hospital, a little over seven months later, on 30 July 1914. At the ensuing coronial, held at the Kew Hospital for the Insane, her death was attributed to arteriosclerosis and insanity.

Though she was described in the doctor's report as Church of England, she was Irish by decent and a Roman Catholic.

I think I got to meet all of the Hobbs females of Mum's generation and I feel I can speak for them: they were anything but bad, like your grandmother, rather strict, judgemental, intolerant and conventional.

I can't imagine any of them running a bad house, though, whatever that may mean!

Good luck with your endeavours.

Uncle Edward

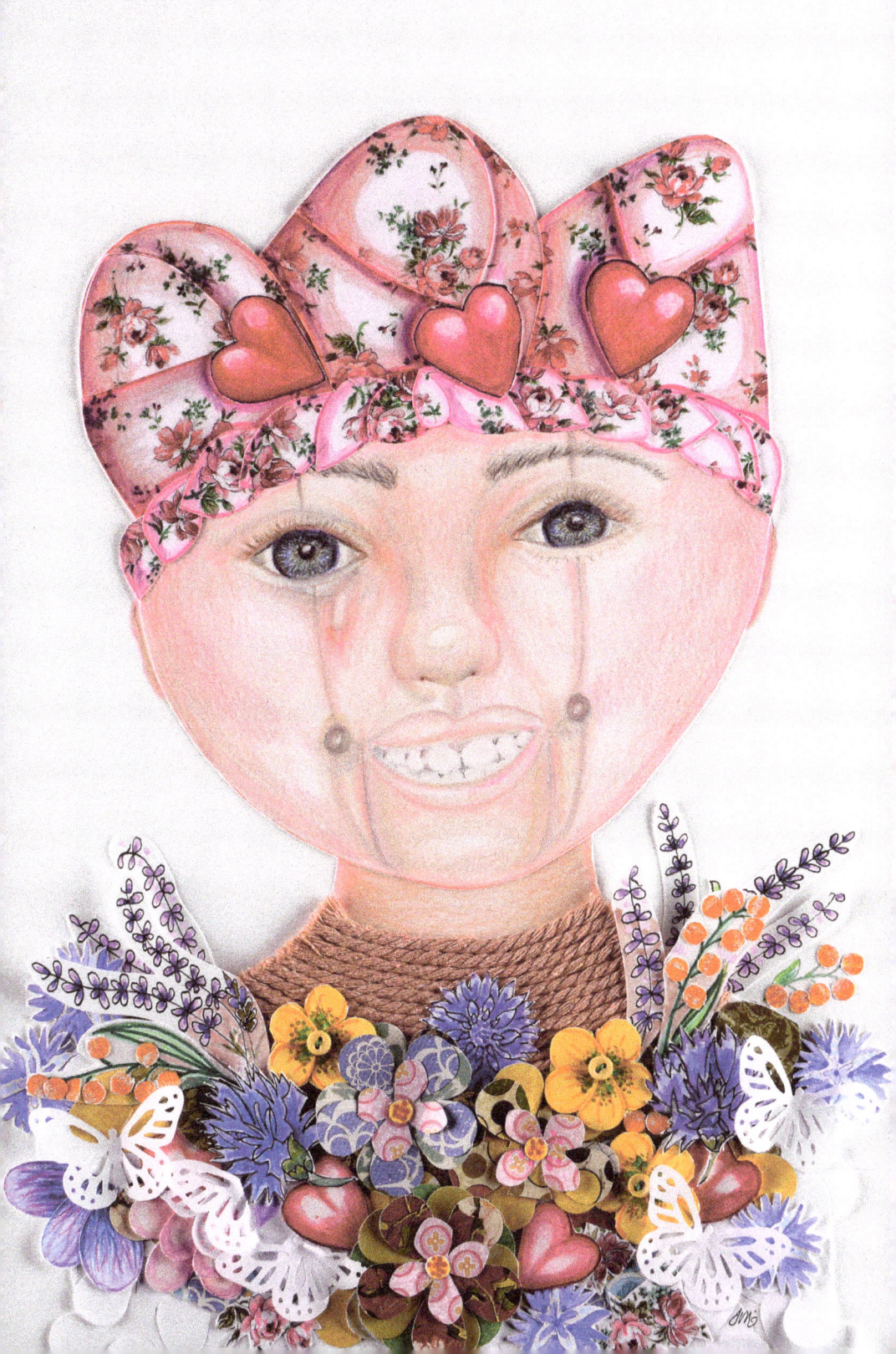

1968

I was born to rusted right-wing, non-feminist parents – they embraced misogyny as though it was a religious calling. Either way, I'd been born on the wrong side of gender from the get-go. My mother was a ringer for a movie star from the golden age of film, Jane Russell. A beautiful, dark-haired fashionista, cordon bleu cook, dedicated homemaker and loyal to my father beyond reproach. My father was street-smart, handsome and a complete charmer of all, but especially other women, unfortunately for my mother. He named me after Jacqueline Kennedy Onassis due to having a major crush on America's First Lady of the time, wholeheartedly viewing her as 'classy'.

I felt that I loved my parents so much I possessed an amazing ability to hold on for dear life to every word that came out their mouths to the point where my fingers would bleed. I didn't have conversations with my parents; well, I did, but only when alcohol was involved, with them drinking, not me. My drinking problem was to occur a bit later.

The house rules were:

1. Only speak when you're spoken to

2. Do as I say, don't do as I do

3. Kids and paint don't mix

4. Keep yourself nice

The first rule I found incredibly difficult to adhere to until I was at least eight. I was a complete failure on rule number two. I broke the third rule when I was four, when I got into my older sister Jane's nail polish collection and pushed my single bed back from the wall. I started expressing my inner Picasso using our seventies monochromatic flocked bedroom wallpaper as a canvas. Rule four was given to me directly by Dad and I had no idea what it meant until I was told on my first day of high school.

'Listen to me and listen good, Jack. If you don't keep yourself nice, you'll get a fat arse, do you understand?'

And no, I had no idea what he was talking about but I nodded anyway. I was raised on tough love and for my siblings I think it worked ok. I, on the other hand, maybe took it too literally.

Here's the problem: from the time I was young, after I'd been smacked or hit or kicked, I'd be reminded by my mother, as she sat on my bed consoling me, rubbing my back to slow my crying, that I was treated that way because they loved me. Speaking softly and smelling of sweet wine, she'd start her speech. It was the same every time.

'Jack, if we didn't smack you, it'd mean we didn't care; we have to show you what's wrong and right and we love you so much. Good night sweetheart.'

My light would go off and, laying in the dark, I'd get to thinking about where I'd gone wrong. How I could be a better person so I wouldn't be smacked or hit or kicked.

The dilemma lay dominantly in the fact that I grew up and took the two words, tough and love, and mixed them with the baseless notion that unless I was being physically ill-treated by those I loved, then I wasn't trying hard enough. Or if I was treated badly by anyone then I had to try harder to gain their love and approval. It was a textbook example of how a child starts to see abuse as appreciation and fondness. Where if she's not experiencing it regularly, life starts to feel very uncomfortable. In turn, she starts to play out because things aren't dramatic enough. But let me set the scene from when my life began or as my father use to phrase it: 'Before you were an itch in my pants'.

My parents were born pre-WW2, around 1930. My mother, who was the youngest child of five, had her life laid out by her father, my grandad Alfred, who in WW1 fought the German attack on Villers-Bretonneux. He returned from the war, was given land by the government to farm and married my Nanna Alma who was ten years his junior at seventeen.

My grandparents were incredibly kind people who, oddly enough, wanted my mother to complete her university degree after she finished teacher's college, but Mum told them was sick of being poor. They wanted her to gain her degree in the field of science; she did too, but also wanted a lifestyle that being a student couldn't provide. My mother was in tears in the weeks leading up to her twenty-fourth birthday. She was sure she'd be left on the shelf, set to become a spinster. Then she met my dad and four months later they were engaged. Once married, the Victorian Education Department released her of her duties as a teacher because married women weren't allowed to have a career. Obviously, the Liberal Party held power at the time.

My father was born the eldest and only son of a good-looking, lovable man, Poppy, and my Nanna Ruby, who had been a nurse in a psychiatric hospital. Ruby didn't have a maternal bone in her body. She grew up in a very small town in Gippsland, Victoria, and made her way into Melbourne very quickly. She was smart and wanted to climb the social ladder but somehow was diverted on her way to Toorak and ended up with Poppy who didn't live anywhere near the overtly affluent suburb.

My family has a history of alcohol dependency, either by it earning them a living or by drinking the products off the shelf. From humble beginnings, my great-grandfather George owned three hotels across regional Victoria in the early 1870s and was so profitable that it allowed them to own a holiday house in Hawthorn within Melbourne's inner eastern suburbs. It was from these taverns that I'm sure Poppy had his first drink and learned from a very early age where you could go to get one or five, for that matter. Dad was also introduced to drink from a very young age at the same pubs.

I was launched into alcohol dependency very subtly at home from the age of six when Dad proudly showed me how to pour a beer. He would give me the last sip before I was to return to the fridge to refill his glass. Standing on a chair to reach the bench, I'd pour the cold liquid from an amber, long-neck Melbourne Bitter bottle. If there was too much in his favourite Shield Abbey goblet for me to carry back, I drank the overflowing foam top then proudly returned the glass to him.

To say I had a predisposition to alcohol would be an understatement. Dad said you could always find Poppy at the local pub, and Nanna Ruby often sent him to drag Poppy home. He had also been blessed with the looks of a movie star; think Leonardo DiCaprio. He was a born womaniser too. A true Peter Pan archetype. Unfortunately, when Poppy roamed, Nanna became extremely volatile and took it out on Dad. The physical abuse started when he was a very small boy. Eventually Nanna and Poppy split up, but never divorced. They just lived in different residences: Poppy on his farm in the Gippsland district and Nanna Ruby in Melbourne. It was then that my dad was bestowed with being the main male role model of the house. He lived with Ruby and his younger sister, my Aunt Brandy. Dad also grew up with the characteristics of both his parents, as you do. He was a very charismatic man with business smarts and the social skills of a politician. Back then violence within the family was never questioned, it just was. There was not a psychologist, counsellor or 24/7 helpline in sight.

In our family home on an average night, ten minutes before Dad was due home, I was ordered by Mum to go wash my face, brush my hair and put on a clean top to make myself 'look pretty' for him. Mum would put on a 'fresh face' of make-up.

'Oh, and don't forget to put on a big smile.'

'OK.'

'OK isn't a word. What do you say?'

'Yes, Mum.'

I'd make a quick exit to the bathroom to find a face washer then start scrubbing the dirt off my face, arms and legs to look presentable.

'Jack, run out and greet your father as he gets out of the car, carry his bag in for him too. He's had a long day. And what are you going to do?'

'Smile.'

'Good girl. Go.'

I had a wardrobe full of pretty dresses and shiny patent leather shoes even though I much preferred hanging out with my cocker spaniel Robyn or in a huge plum tree in our large garden in my dirty overalls and my favourite green plastic cowboy hat. I was a tomboy at heart. Bee stings were a common event as I chose to roll down our sloping block into piles of pine-scented sawdust, and even though I was allergic to bees the fun outweighed the pain and swelling of my feet and hands. Mum's remedy was to remove the sting with a pair of tweezers then soak the infected body part in boiling water mixed with bleach. It was my mother who thought bleach fixed everything, well before Donald Trump ever did.

When I look back I can see my willingness to look after the men in my life came from watching and mirroring Mum in the way she looked after Dad. Unfortunately, no matter how much she looked after him and pleased him, he still behaved terribly. The worse he behaved the harder she tried – a vicious cycle. She prepared all the meals, laid out all his clothes on the bed including his underwear, polished shoes, and cleaned the house until it shone – the lot. I remember shoving rubbish in my jean pockets because I couldn't use the bins as she'd scrubbed them until they were spotless. She'd then tell me off when she did the laundry. I would hear her screaming from the laundry.

'Jack! Oh my God, why have you got rubbish in your pockets?'

I'd run and hide in a tree, being at a loss for where to put the rubbish!

On an average night, my brother and I would hear taunts from Dad of how hopeless and stupid we were. That was often the last thing we would hear before we went to sleep. There were good nights but they were rare because we never knew how the alcohol would influence Dad's mood.

That was the privileged family I grew up with, perfect from the outside, literally. A white, picture-perfect, storybook house surrounded by a large brick wall and ornate, wrought iron gates. We had beautiful gardens and open land with a pool and tennis court, but behind closed doors it could become extremely dysfunctional and ugly.

I was bestowed with the talent of masking my face with happiness from a very young age. When I wore the mask, it was perfect to those who saw me, even my older siblings. I felt as though I always had to be on show. I had to be happy with everything and everybody, constantly nodding and smiling.

Eventually it was my job to look pretty, stay skinny, and be humourous but not funny, as that would make me a show-off. I was never to forget the first rule: only speak when you're spoken to. I wasn't raised to have an opinion. When asked by friends or strangers what my opinion was even as an adult I normally fell in a nervous heap, as being in agreement with others was safer. My favourite rule was to be safe and stay between the lines. Other children who could be so-called 'naughty' would send me into a compete panic; I was horrified to think what their dads would do to them.

There were endless times when Dad was drunk and would coax me to sit down, as he wanted to talk. He'd take interest in my dreams and daily happenings, or so I thought. In the morning, he wouldn't have the slightest recollection of our conversation, so I became very confused as to why he wasn't interested in continuing the discussions from the night previous. To me the fear he projected was all-consuming. I wanted us to have a relationship that I knew my other girlfriends had with their fathers. I could never make Dad happy though, no matter how hard I tried. The more I tried, the more it pushed him away.

I have to remember he was a man uncomfortable with affection from his family, but being admired and held in high regard from strangers was something he valued much more than his wife or children.

I was born a pleaser, so when Dad lost his temper, I would follow him, constantly calling out his name and making a bad situation worse for myself. He would turn to see me following him, crying. Calling out his name made him break into a run. He would yell at me to fuck off – not that I knew what that meant, but I knew he was angry.

I held onto that. I made it my job to make sure those around me were happy and smiling, or at least I gave it my best shot. It was a feeling that ran through most of my adult life; I had to get people to like me. I loved everyone so it was only fair they reciprocated.

One night, I wasn't even two, my parents had guests over for one of their infamous dinner parties. I recall Mum holding me in her arms and then handing me over to one of the male guests at the gathering. He held me in his hands, broadly smiling, arms outstretched. Then he started bouncing me. Next thing, he threw me up in the air and caught me, which I must have thought was great fun. But then he got bit too enthusiastic. He threw me up to the ceiling, hitting my head on a wrought iron chandelier. My hair got caught on a turned hook within the light fixture. It was the strangest sound, then a piercing pain. I felt warmth running down my head. I burst into tears. I remember being unable to catch my breath after screaming. Dad yelled at Mum to get me out of the room and, before I knew it, I was in my cot being yelled at for making a scene. The door quickly shut on me; I sobbed myself to sleep. I distinctly recall thinking that my head was hurting but I was confused and scared. I had red on my hands and dress. Fifty years later, when I asked Mum if I recalled that event correctly, she said I had. I'd been bleeding from my scalp where I'd lost a piece of my hair to the metal hook. I remember distinctly feeling guilty. It was bizarre. I felt it was my fault.

It's something I've been able to do since I was very young, precisely recall events. I'm not talking about stories that have been told about me through my mother and siblings so often they have become my reality. I'm talking about incidents that occurred when I was a baby that I can vividly recall, where points of reference all add up to a pattern and I can see my childhood made of moments that are poignant, such as when I fell out of a window.

My parents were near the final stages of building our family home. My father helped build it on the weekends so we'd all get bundled into the new, pale green American Dodge he'd bought from the proceeds of a successful business he and Mum had built. We all headed off, 1970s style, no seat belts, driving to our two-acre block, 35 kilometres outside of Melbourne. I was wearing navy corduroy overalls over a cream woollen hand-knitted jumper, as it was a cool and cloudy day. I was in Dad's arms and he was talking to our builder, Mr Strachan. Dad would remind anyone who asked about the house that Mr Strachan was the father of Shirley Strachan, lead singer of the famous 1970s Melbourne rock band Skyhooks. They were laughing and Dad

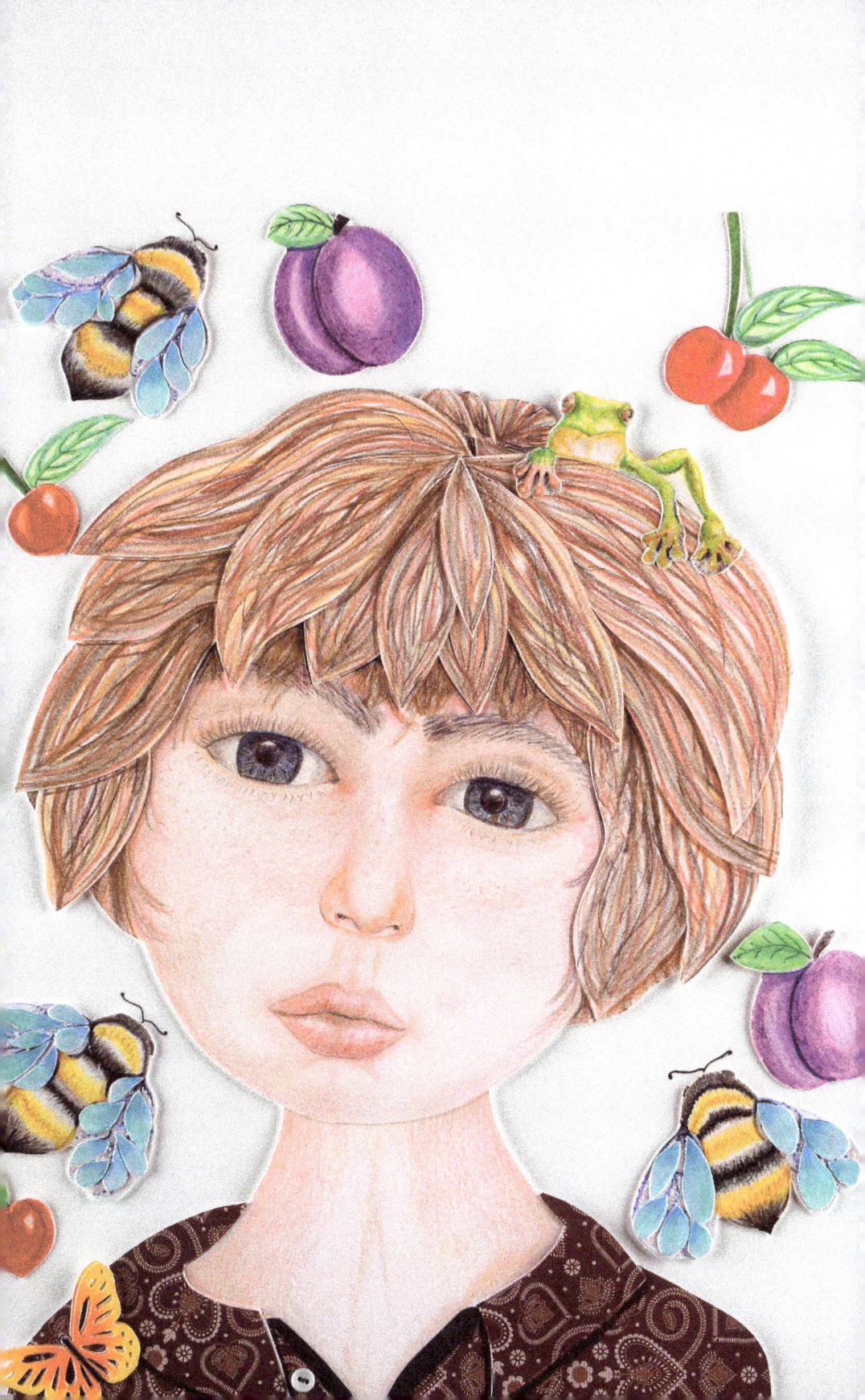

turned and sat me on a window ledge – the bathroom window facing east, to be exact. He left me balancing on the ledge, which was approximately 180 centimetres off the ground. I wasn't scared, I was just happy I could see things, as I was higher than I would have been at ground level. It didn't take long until I was free falling. Then my head was hurting, my body too. Dad yelled at Mum.

'Come and get her. Put her inside, she's making a scene!'

What I can visualise is being told over and over to stop crying, my mother jiggling me. I was in terrible pain and she wasn't making it better by bouncing me up and down, go figure. Then the recollection ends. The exact scenario was confirmed by Mum a few years ago. She couldn't believe I was even able to tell her what I wore that day, let alone the weather.

It's one of many superpowers I possess. The first is bipolar, which is my strongest superpower. It will never win me a Nobel Peace Prize but it's fun at family gatherings – the clothes and weather superpower, not the bipolar one. The bipolar one tends to send friend and foe running away from me when activated, but more on that later. When I dream it's incredibly vivid too. I can recall events in dreams that I may have had years previously. I can still recall dreams I experienced as a child.

1972

From a very early age I'd learned that if I couldn't make Dad laugh with a joke, if I couldn't 'butter him up', it could be a terrible night ahead. I would do nearly anything when he'd been drinking to cajole him because I never knew how the evening would turn out. Sitting on his lap and hugging him, kissing his face, giggling – just anything to make him smile – always on the ready to respond and fix situations that had been blown out of proportion, to calm, to sooth, to pacify. If that didn't work, I found places to hide. It was a game I played with myself as a child. *Where could I fit that a big person couldn't?* I'd even time myself. How could I roll into a ball and calm my breathing so a big person couldn't detect me? All I had to do was close my eyes and I'd disappear. Breathe slowly, calm down, disappear. I even tried to jump into the pages of the book I'd laid out on my bedroom floor, Mary Poppins style. Only one problem: if I got in how was I going to get out? I could visualise Dad violently shaking it as though willing me to fall out onto the ground below.

'You little shit, get out of the book now or I will bloody kill you!'

Then Mum: 'Jack, sweetie, listen to your father, he's not kidding. Look for the nearest door. That's a door that leads outside, not inside, not an internal door.'

Note to self: do not jump in the book.

To say I was overly anxious would be an understatement. Even today if I'm around certain men I will become extremely nervous. It's almost like sensing male dominance within a confined space. I have to be very aware that I don't give away that which is rightfully mine, a space to be myself. To me it means to be solid in my conviction of who I am and not to waver or be pressured otherwise.

I wasn't raised with a true sense of self. I had no idea who I was, what I stood for or where I belonged. I couldn't pick up a self-help book and have everything fall into place. If I took an interest in a hobby or tried to learn a new skill, Dad had a habit of popping his head around the corner and making snide remarks at me that I was a show-off. I was removed from many after-school classes, not long after making new friends. He hated being overshadowed. I believe it is why I learned not to trust my instincts and was constantly changing my mind, doing anything to avoid getting into trouble. Even from primary school age, being invited to parties as a little girl would send me into such an anxious state an hour prior to going, as I always had this feeling he would turn up and abruptly pull me away from playing with the other kids.

There were times as an adult when I would accept invitations to events only to fall into a heap before going due to nerves. I felt like a fraud, like I wasn't good enough to go. I had a habit of drinking a lot in public when I was asked to places. I knew that alcohol could drown all my fears and yet inflate a false sense of self. It was a work in progress trying to balance quantity and accountability.

Some people love food or coffee; I loved alcohol. That doesn't mean I was a connoisseur, it means I loved the feeling it gave me: both confidence and a sense of floating, of being underwater. It's the soft golden reflection of the wine, still or sparkling, inside an elegant, blown glass, glistening with tenacity and spirit, literally. By the second glass I was always in another dimension.

Unfortunately, with Dad alcohol made his already sober solid sense of self blow out of proportion, and he'd turn into a fierce oppressor, madly squashing those around him as though we were invasive bugs.

My best friend Clair was staying at my house after school one Friday night for a sleep over when we were fourteen. We had everything organised: a video (it was the early eighties) and snacks. It was around 8 pm when Dad completely lost it. Clair and I still don't recall why but he flew into the family room, enraged. Mum was ordered to call Clair's mum Eve who lived forty-five minutes away. I was terribly humiliated and crushed. Clair can explain it from her perspective still now.

'I never forget what he did during that first year. I was verbally attacked by your father in your home, accused of being a dangerous influence and unworthy of your association and was ordered to phone my parents for immediate collection. He insisted that we cut ties and that I must never darken your doorstep again. My utter shock and horror at this is an understatement still now. His words and rage made me feel shamed but I did not know why, while your mother silently watched on. After this, I became more aware of the toll this volatile and unpredictable environment had on you. I also wanted to help support and strengthen you as best a fourteen-year-old can. My loving family helped too, making it clear that you were always welcome, safe and immensely valued.'

Clair's family pretty much adopted me. They became my second home; they loved me so much. It was a huge comfort for me to be surrounded by people who accepted me no matter what. It was there I learned so much: what was wrong and what was right, what was ugly and what nurturing meant.

I learned very quickly that any words of support from Dad were only bestowed upon me once he was either intoxicated or in front of complete strangers, who would then view him as a good father and proud pillar of the community. He was a senior member of a worldwide charity organisation and rose in the ranks due to his philanthropic endeavours. He made over one million dollars in one of his last money-generating ideas before his retirement, let alone what he made in the forty years of being involved. He was enormously kind to complete strangers, so very big-hearted. To his children though the descriptions he gave my brother and I were normally that along the lines of how dumb and stupid we were: 'Thick as 4x2's' (planks of timber), 'absolutely hopeless' or a 'burden to the whole family'. After being told that time and again, I felt like nothing. I carried a sense of emptiness that couldn't be filled, yet I would keep trying to fill it, even into my adulthood.

I was always thinking in the negative and if something good did happen then it was a bonus – only other people experienced good things. If it was taken away, I didn't expect any better, so I wouldn't be as disappointed; a recipe for black pessimism to sprout within the mind of a child.

From prep onwards I can remember I never really tried reading or engaging in any class activity other than art and drama; I was considered a 'dreamer'. When my first report card from prep arrived, it had Fs all across it. Dad leant down and, looking me straight in the eyes, told me I was a failure and that I may as well give up school there and then. I always panicked when tests came around because it was as though I was looking at another language other than English; it was not unlike a type of Morse code really. There was a constant cloud over my head that no matter what I tried I'd get it wrong because I was told I was a 'half-wit'. Often I only wrote my name on the top of the page, nothing else.

My two older sisters, Anne and Jane, had left home before Dad started to drink heavily and they never incurred any alcohol-fuelled abuse. However, he could still cause grief due to his quick temper. It was his way or the highway. Jane married early in her life to get out of the house. Anne travelled the world and once back in Melbourne she gained a good job that enabled her to live away from home. For me, leaving wasn't an option, so I built my persona on what other people wanted me to be and not on who I really was. Jane jokingly called me a chameleon. Looking back, I lived the life of a different person, or many different people, until I came to a point of exhaustion and stopped; but it took a very long time. On the inside, I just wouldn't grow up and nor did I want to. What I wanted was life to be happy and wonderful and I craved it terribly. I was so fearful of responsibility; it was always something other people had to deal with because I felt everyone else knew better than I did. My life hinged on trying to be pretty, skinny, delightful and, most importantly, agreeable as it was safer. I had this sure sense that I wasn't to be trusted. It was to be to my absolute detriment because I gave away any power I had over my young life.

1982 – March

A major turning point in my life occurred one evening when I was sitting in the family room watching TV with my brother Alex. Mum came into the room with a few drinks under her multi-coloured polyester kaftan and asked us in her most charming air hostess voice if we would like a drink of milk and a biscuit. We took up the offer, sat down at the burnt orange linoleum breakfast bar and started consuming our treat. Enter Dad. All I remember was being yelled at by him to get to bed as he slapped the doorframe as hard as he could with his brown leather slipper. Immediately, Mum told us to hurry up and drink the milk. Trying to please both of them, I panicked, shoved the whole biscuit in my mouth and drank the milk to a point where I couldn't fit anymore into my mouth. I got out of my chair and ran, quickly following Alex up the hall. I can clearly visualise Dad coming after us, yelling verbal abuse, trying to get us to move faster.

'Fucking move, you little bastards.'

At that moment, I felt a blunt painful force in my lower back and, as I lunged forward from losing my footing, I sprayed milk and biscuit all over the wall and carpet. I landed face first on the floor, carpet grazing my chin. I would later learn that Dad had kicked me in the tailbone, my coccyx.

Now both Alex and I knew we were really in for it. Dad picked me up by my shoulders and threw me into my bedroom. I landed head first against the windows. Thank goodness the thick curtains were drawn and the panes of glass were small so the force of my impact only cracked one. Slamming my bedroom door and shutting me in my room alone, he then started on my brother. From the banging sounds heard, I imagined that Dad had pushed Alex into his wardrobe doors and was hitting him with clenched fists. He was yelling at Alex over and over.

'You are a fucking stupid boy.'

I couldn't stand being hit or yelled at but, even more so, I couldn't handle my brother having it happen to him. I was younger than Alex by five years. We were never close growing up but I felt I had to protect him. I opened my bedroom door and ran into my brother's room, trying hysterically to wedge myself between my father's fists and my brother's body. Dad hit me instead, leaving a bruise on my neck and shoulder. I had so much anxiety running through my veins I wanted to take the whole impact of it, all of it.

Mum eventually turned up and pulled Dad off Alex and me, but the damage had been done. My brother was bleeding and cowering on his bedroom floor.

Later, once we had all retreated into our closed rooms, I clearly recall hearing Mum yell at Dad at the top of her voice.

'If you ever hit me, I swear to God, I will leave you and you'll have nobody.'

The next day she told me that she'd never leave him, and asked why would she. I shouldn't have been surprised because, when I was four, she told me that Dad would always come first in her life, even above my brother, me and my sisters. He was her husband and that's what made a family.

I felt alone, unprotected and betrayed even though I couldn't verbalise it. The main male figure in my life that I looked up to and loved scared me to death. I loved him but I hated him too. After all the commotion and things settling down, my only thought was that maybe I wasn't trying hard enough to love him.

But the woman who I also looked up to and held so close to my heart, my mum, had let my brother and I down too, which hurt even more. I never felt wanted and it was something I carried through most of my adult life, which in return made me needy.

Mum always got Dad to say sorry at breakfast after he'd been on a bender the previous night. It was never a clear apology though; he never looked at me when he said it, mumbling under his voice. It was always a sheepish attempt.

I went to school the day after the incident for my year eight class photo, my eyes puffed up and red from crying all night and not sleeping out of fear. I turned up my school collar to cover the welt on my neck only to have it turned down by the photographer when the pictures were taken. I prayed he wouldn't see anything or mention it if he did; but back then people never mentioned anything even if they did notice.

The pain in my back was excruciating and the damage would eventually lead to major surgery two years later and a disk being removed from my spine.

A small gift from Mum was on my bed when I got home from school, as it always was after a night of abuse. You've heard of a 'push present' for delivering a baby. Well, this was the 'sorry souvenir' for taking the abuse, a peace offering, one of many over the years. But she never sincerely apologised until I was forty-five. From Dad I received nothing nor ever heard a word.

On many occasions, I had the privilege (or so they thought) of being told wise and important things by my parents. They would make it sound like I was the luckiest person in the world because they were divulging this information to me. With bated breath I would wait for words that would come out of their mouths that I knew would change the game plan.

Let me set the scene for you. I was in the family room. Mum popped her head through the door to tell me to come into the lounge room. Read: adults only area, children must be invited in. She politely told me to sit down.

'Now, your father and I have been talking and I saw a notice in your school bag that said you're about to start your work experience over the next two weeks and you need to pick two jobs. Have you had any thoughts, darling?'

I started to tell her I wanted to be a Qantas air hostess, but Dad put the kibosh on that.

'You won't be able to cope being away from home and all you'll be doing is picking up peoples chuck bags.'

OK, one down. Before I could express any other aspirations though, Mum jumped in.

'Sweetie, we're thinking retail'.

Ah ... not what I had in mind but, anyway, what would I know?

'You would suit that, sweetie. You just have to stand there, smile and look, well, pretty. I mean, really, you won't have to worry about a career, darling, that's for girls who are clever and who aren't going to get married. You'll be fine. You'll meet a nice boy one day and he'll sweep you off your feet and look after you for the rest of your life.'

My mind snapped, a new lesson noted: a man will look after me. I'd be dependent on another man. No argument. Which man I had no idea, but I'd find one, as that's what was expected.

'In the meantime, listen to our guidance, follow everything we tell you to do and you'll be fine … OK? Good girl. You can go now.'

I can clearly look back at that time and recall my girlfriends in high school gaining work experience in the most amazing companies, doing incredible things. I didn't have the confidence to step out from my parents' navigation nor did my parents have the confidence in me to be able to step away and allow me to make choices, be they wrong or right.

Marriage seemed to always be the answer my parents gave me to quite a few of my questions growing up. Pity they didn't have a crystal ball because to date I do not have a great track record with matrimony. Every year their wedding anniversary came around, and every year Mum crooned the same comments when I asked her how she was about meeting the milestone.

'Sweetie, did you know this year will be our sixtieth wedding anniversary? The funny thing is, you wouldn't get that for bloody murder and I don't know what I did wrong in my past life to deserve it.'

They also claimed they both deserved a medal. I suppose it should be called a millstone, not a milestone. That way they could hang the medal proudly around their necks. Not too tightly though, I hope, it could do some damage. I wouldn't want that now … would I?

1980s

Genealogy. Your lineage. Your family tree. It can evoke inquisitive enthusiasm within many a person like nothing you've ever witnessed. I never used to understand why it enthralled people so much.

A recent visit to Clair's mother's for a cup of tea became an hour-long session inquisitively looking at stained, musty photos and council documents dating back to the late 1800s in Melbourne, all spread across her antique dining room table. I didn't necessarily want to pinpoint a place of origin; mine was a search for health reasons. I wanted to know why I was so different from my family. As in, vastly different. My behaviour at times, well, it was just off.

I had so many unanswered questions. Why, at fourteen, after a bottle of Blackberry Nip at a friend's party, did I decide to jump from the roof into the pool? Why was I the girl hanging out of train doors by my fingers just to feel the wind push over my body as I rolled with the movement, pushing myself to let go as the train caught up speed? I became high on risk. Why did I have such a heightened sense of sexuality that stayed with me into adulthood, playing out to a point where my sister and her husband threatened to remove my son due to a life choice of wanting become a prostitute? I experienced waves of wanting to go shopping, rampantly entering every shop and putting thousands of dollars on a credit card Dad had given me, purchasing anything that I thought someone I knew would like. I'd return home with bags upon bags of goods that covered my bed and flooded the floor of my room. I'd lose sleep over what I'd done, only to return the items the next day in a rush of panic. I both loathed and loved that feeling.

In the summer of 1986, my girlfriends and I headed down to Sorrento in Melbourne's bayside to stay at my uncle's holiday house. We headed to the pub to celebrate. Once there I decided to shout the bar – the entire bar.

It was a brilliant night of drinking to excess; I drank everything available, including a leftover stubby with cigarettes butts in it. My final act, just after we were kicked out at closing time, was to stand at the top of the steep stairs, all thirty plus of them, which lead to the main street. I stood, staring down, then fell into a free fall, tumbling over and over all the way to the cold concrete below. I made it to the bottom amazed that I'd finally stopped. I jumped up as though I was the greatest circus act on Earth. There was a stunned silence from my newly gathered audience, then came the magical uproar – it was brilliant. I made a great number of friends that night that I was never to come across again.

The fall ended with me in bed the following day. Two dislocated fingers, body terribly bruised and enormously hungover, vomiting continually until the following evening. God, it was so worth it!

During university, I often paid for long lunches with five, ten, fifteen classmates – well, my folks were. It excited me; generosity gave me a thrill like no other. I couldn't understand why my parents refused to understand that I was making others happy because of my generosity—I mean, their benevolence.

The tables had finally turned. I was now stealing money out of my father's wallet. It was palpable, this intense need to please my friends. I knew it was wrong, I have a conscience, but in all honesty, I never saw being physically, verbally and emotionally mistreated as 'something out of the ordinary'. I just felt he owed me, both of them owed me, and I was spending on people who appreciated me. They loved me because I was the fun one. I was the needy one and they took, but it felt so right. To take risks, financial hits that brought elevated highs then turmoil – it was my drug. I never needed cocaine, heroin or methamphetamine. I had something much better, and it cost me nothing but my pride. I gambled with my life constantly. I took big risks when no one was watching or when everyone was watching it was even a bigger rush. Dare me, or don't dare me, I didn't care; I'd still do it.

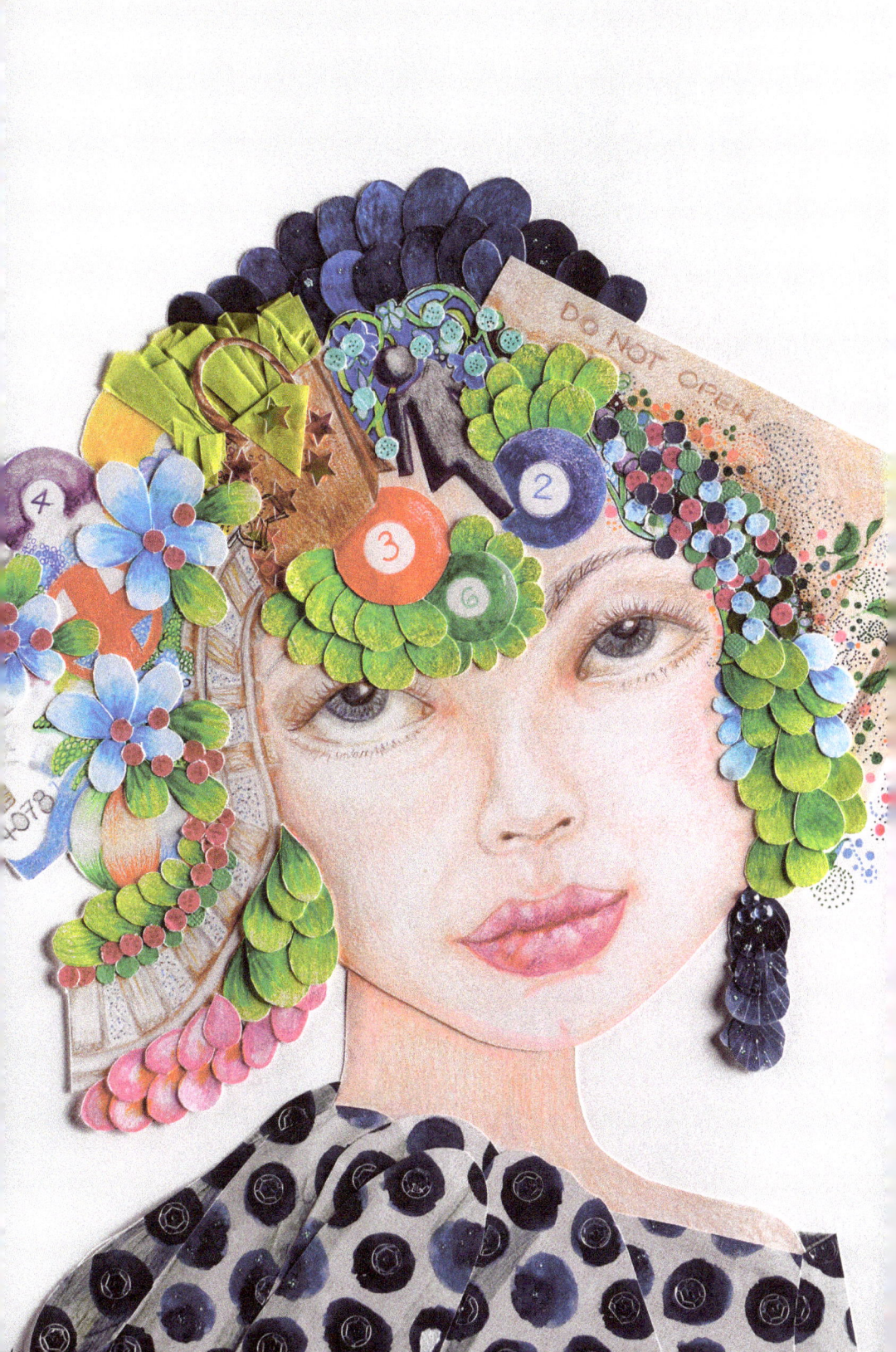

It was an exuberant feeling, a bewitching potion that ran through every cell in my body, lifting me to a higher plane, closer to God. He spoke to me too, loud and clear. Metaphysical jabber in my mind, words, talking, disagreements, never stopping, over and over. I could reach the stars, be bigger than the world, a universe full of glitter, entirely enthralling. I'd consume everything my mind could take and then I'd tire and it would stop. Thick black mud would enter my space, overwhelming my entire soul. My magic disappeared again; my crystal glass that was full of pure raging ego now was empty. I'd exhale into exhausted paranoia, roll up into a ball, into nothing. Days on end in bed were to follow, a bankruptcy of self, a shocking sense of embarrassment. I'd fucked up again and again. Repetitive, screaming insanity. I'd scratch at my scalp, making it bleed, my skin crawling with cockroaches. It was like the drinks cupboard had a banner above it stating, 'In case of emergency, drink to the stop the voices'. And I drank.

At forty-three, after twenty-one different antidepressant medications it finally had a name. I needed to know that I wasn't the only one in my family who felt like this. I needed to be shown why.

I sat opposite a new psychiatrist, my fifth to date, and he said he had the answer.

'Jackie, I believe you've been misdiagnosed over the years. You have bipolar, bipolar 2. It's not any less worse than being bipolar 1, it's really a number to differentiate it.'

He waited for my reply.

I remember quietly whispering in reply, deadpan and empty. I was drained of energy again. 'That's definitely me; I'm different.'

'Do you know if any another family member has it? Maybe a history within your family?'

'I don't know. I'd have to check ancestry.com.'

I didn't mean to be a smart arse; I was just over all the drama.

1970s

From my first day entering the public school system in prep at aged five, I loathed it. I cried for the first two weeks. I missed Mum so much it hurt. My brother Alex was being taught at the same school but never checked on me. Not due to any malice, but rather that it wasn't seen as cool. With that, as well as the fact that those who cried a lot were picked on, school was horrendous.

It was and still is a part of Darwin's theory of evolution: a dog-eat-dog mentality. Every morning brought on a feeling of panic that could not be justified, so I still had to attend school with the heels of my Mary Jane's digging in the dirt.

By the time secondary school came around I was well and truly feeling the unease of what only teen hormones can bring on. My best friend at the time, who I really didn't like because she was an absolute know-it-all princess, spent most weekends attending kiddy beauty pageants. I justifiably felt ugly and completely out of place next to her. Her name: Elizabeth. Mum even signed me up to do kiddie gym classes with her, but, as she was far more graceful and elegant than I, that seemed in my head to give her greater power over me. To this day I still shudder thinking about other kids starry-eyed mothers applying hideous blue eye shadow on my irritated lids and sticky leg tan that left a stain on Mum's good Egyptian cotton bed sheets.

Why befriend someone you couldn't stand? I hear you ask. Well, I had an unconscious understanding with myself that if I kept the most popular, bitchy girl in school close by then I wouldn't endure her wrath as much as if I wasn't her friend. It was how I viewed my relationship with my dad coincidently. Better the devil you know, as Kylie sings.

So with the primary school beauty queen beside me, I started to encounter what are normal teenage goings-on. Enter oily skin, pubic hair and my first period, something I was never told about. I innocently walked into the school toilets before heading home on my bike and then it hit me fair in the head. I was staring down at blood on my knickers thinking, *Oh my God, I'm dying!* I wasn't, but the maternal power that was my mother forgot to inform me that something would happen at about age twelve. I got home and all she could do was hand me a thick sanitary napkin. What to do with it, I didn't have the faintest.

'Here, use this. You're not going to die.'

As an added bonus, I was given an introduction to sex education the same night when I'd just turned off the light to go to sleep. Dad knocked on my door, walking into my bedroom.

'Move over,' he said.

I obliged.

Lying next to me on top of the covers, he said the following: 'Jack, don't sleep around with boys or you'll get a fat ass. I've told you since you were a whippet: keep yourself nice. Night.'

He got up, exited my room and that was it, thus ending the sex education talk. So that's what he meant by 'keep yourself nice'.

I would lie in bed for hours staring at the ceiling and praying to God that I wouldn't get pregnant. I didn't know that you had to partake in the physical act of intercourse – I just thought if a boy liked you and looked at you for too long it would happen.

Just when I was thinking surely things couldn't get any more embarrassing for me as a post-pubescent teen, I found out very abruptly that when your mum is driving you to the local high school in a luxury car you are bound to stand out.

Enter Cheryl, a very angry and aggressive girl the same age as me who'd been raised in the local caravan park in the next suburb. I knew of her from her previous actions of putting a packet of laxatives in the scone dough that we were making in home economics class. If she sat behind you in class you could be assured you would have either chewing gum in your hair by the end of the lesson or a lock of your hair missing, cut off by the knife she kept in her pocket. She scared the living crap out of me and that was half my problem. My fear was obviously sensed, not unlike a hungry bull shark sensing a Maltese puppy paddling in a Gold Coast canal. She'd taken a shining to me that I hadn't noticed, but let's just say it wasn't a secret crush of good tiding; I think the word stalking would describe it best. She had an uncanny habit of standing against my locker so I couldn't gain access to it, willing me to ask her to please move. And, boy, did I fix her good and proper. I went to many of my classes with none of the books.

One afternoon though, when the final bell rang, I ran over to the bike rack with Elizabeth, grabbed my two-wheeled mode of transport and started my way home. I was no further out the school gate when, just as I mounted my seat and started peddling, Cheryl, who was standing at the bus shelter, lurched forward towards me. I heard her make a noise, which was that of her sucking air deeply through her nose and gathering mucus from her air passages. She then spat on my face. I fell off my bike from the shock that I had been officially slagged on.

'Take that, snooty. Where's mummies car when you need it? Fucking bitch!'

I was then kicked in the ribs and all the kids who witnessed it just laughed, including Elizabeth. I was bruised and gutted, literally and metaphorically speaking. When I finally peddled home with bruised ribs, grazed hands and knees, as well an embarrassed and heavy heart, I told Mum and she exploded. Ironically, I found this astounding. Dad could kick and hit me and she didn't flinch but she was furious that someone outside the family did.

Now I don't know if you're familiar with astrological terms, but Mum was born in late October and is a Scorpio. The next day when she drove up to the school, all hell broke loose as she channelled her inner arachnid. I may have been in class on the other side of the quadrangle to the headmaster's office but what I heard was scary. The sound was like the roar of a lion – Leo – crossed with charging of a bull – Taurus. From what Mum told me, our school's principal looked like he'd been slapped across the face with two fish – Pisces – and was backing away from her like he had goat's horns rammed up his ass – that would be Capricorn in Uranus.

In her triumphant speech, she told him that his school was not good enough for her daughter, she really should have checked with the school she was sending me to first as they were willing to accept me and she was taking me out immediately … but not for four months. Thank goodness Cheryl was expelled and accepted by another local school closer to her home, but the news was out with my school mates. Thanks to Mum's screeching banshee voice, they had heard their school wasn't good enough, so I was heading over to the local private school. The remaining sixteen weeks were lonelier than ever and even Elizabeth didn't want to be my friend anymore. I was officially over the public school system and ready to cross over to what they all considered to be the dark side.

1982-1984

I adored my new school. At this stage I would like to say that I was given the opportunity to expand my mind beyond any mathematical or literary comprehension, but it wasn't my strongest point at that stage in life. My strength laid in being able to appreciate the aesthetics, the surrounds, the buildings; to me, it was a beautiful retreat from what I was used to. The classrooms had huge widows that framed the surrounding bush land, heated flooring and soft pastel hues painted on the walls. These were newly built architecturally designed buildings where graffiti was not an option and there was a cute little outside chapel up the back of the acreage property. I never attended a religious ceremony there but I did fall to my knees and pray there once to help save my life, but not until 1984.

No, I used the size of the land to embark on my newly found vice for smoking cigarettes stolen from Mum's handbag. Anne had just returned from Paris and had given Mum a packet; they were multi-coloured and gold tipped. There was nothing cooler to this fourteen-year-old than handing out stolen cigarettes to new friends, and it made me happy too. I now had contraband to cajole them with, as I felt I couldn't possibly do it just as myself, empty-handed. It was an offering of sorts, a real conversation starter. I knew in no time word would spread. I may have been the new kid at school but I was cool and I was so desperate to be accepted it was lucky for Mum I couldn't fit her twelve-litre Coolabah wine cask in my backpack.

I desperately wanted to sing our school anthem proudly every Monday morning at assembly, but I didn't want to look too enthusiastic. I ended up just humming it in my mind whilst hanging my head. It was my eagerness in class though that got me sitting next to my future BFF Clair, and here's her version.

'My earliest memory of you was day one of year eight, when, as a new student to the school, you were making quite an impression on the class with the regularity and vigour of your right arm, responding to every question the teacher asked. We all wondered who was this strange creature? I think the teacher did too. It still brings a smile to my face. Perhaps you thought this was what was expected at this school. It was certainly not the typical teenage approach, but given that you looked like a cool chick and seemed friendly, I was curious to find out more about you. I quickly discovered your tremendous observational wit, which had me laughing from that first recess and forever after. Some other charms I soon became aware of were your kindness to all, huge heart, insightful mind and your sparkly spirit, that shone through your eyes.

'Our friendship grew and although we were part of a wider circle of girls and boys there was just a special connection that we shared. We became more like each other so that we often sensed the others' internal currents and could gauge what would be said next. Despite this bond, it was a while until I understood the mental and emotional load you carried daily.'

See, my grades had improved by leaps and bounds, as I felt it was such a nurturing environment that I had entered. I couldn't wipe the smile off my face. My teacher decided I was such a delight he sat me next to the 'rebellious' girl in class, Clair. He obviously thought my imprint would magically wipe off on her like a good case of hair lice. It didn't; his plan backfired.

It was around this time that Dad kicked me up the hallway. A time when I was exposed to domestic violence in all its glory, where he had crossed the line from what was once just an 'acceptable' smack across my legs to show me right from wrong. It happened halfway through my first semester in year eight and I had been achieving A and B plus reports across the board in my studies.

For the first time in my young life, I loved school and was flourishing but after that night a slow decline began even though I had pushed the event to the back of my mind. I found myself becoming internally angry after that night.

Meeting Clair, though, was a monumental moment in my life. It was a huge shock and adventure meeting a girl of the same age that had been raised the complete opposite to myself. I was in awe of her. She was cool, calm and seemed fully in control of her life. Her parents raised her to have a mind and a voice, something I'd never come across in a girl before. I found her courage fascinating but could never mimic it no matter how hard I tried. She was such a breath of fresh air, whereas I was slowly gasping for breath at home. It was shocking.

It was in year nine, aged fifteen, that I started to play out my fuelled anger via using ill humour to put teachers down, even if ever so slightly. I started to get my laughs at the cost of other students that were achieving higher scores; outwardly I hated them, but inwardly I envied them and wanted to be them. By the end of the year I was physically attacking myself by ramming my fists into lockers. Once I got to school, I would start disrupting the class to a point where I would be sent outside to calm down. Now, I ask you, how can a kid calm down if they never saw their parents calm down? I never knew. I didn't even know I had a problem. I would feel this anger welling up inside me. I'd get up from my chair, walk out to my locker, clench my fist up into a tight ball and then smash it into the cold grey metal, over and over again.

Hurting myself felt like an outlet, and I would swing a punch to the point of making my knuckles swell and bleed. The bloodier and more swollen the better. Calm would then come over me and eventually I would return to the classroom, but unable to write because my hand was so inflamed. Mum never questioned why my hands were so wounded.

'What the hell have you done? Don't answer that, just go and wash up.' She sounded weary.

Mum was a trained teacher so when I returned home she would launch on me to do homework as soon as I had finished afternoon tea. Unfortunately though, I saw it as a time to sit at the dining table and read a Dolly magazine whilst filing my nails as the table I was designated was in another room to the kitchen. Instead I'd draw intricate designs of houses, fashion and flowers. Fortunately, there weren't any lockers at home and Mum thought I never tried learning anything at school so I had taken it upon myself to not try at all.

My class attendance got diverted from normal maths to B-maths. It was known as the class for thick kids. Instead of being taught to speak French, I was taught how to cook French recipes and I was never interested in food other than eating it to survive. A running joke with my sisters now is that I use my oven as a sock draw. If my son Angus ever wants me to bake, I must remember to remove the woollens first.

Mum didn't understand what the hell was going on with my grades and renamed me a 'lazy bitch', so I did what any kid would do in that instance. I decided if that's what they called me, then that's what I'd become. I stopped trying altogether. I bounced through life with my main aim to just be funny and get a laugh out of people – that was it. The ability to consciously make people laugh at my expense meant that I had something going for me at least. I then gave too much energy to what other people thought of me – good or, more often than not, bad, depending on the type of humour I used. I unconsciously concluded I didn't have any worth so my attitude came out as though I couldn't care less about learning, didn't give a shit, but I was completely lost as to who I was meant to be. I was as my father would label me: dumb as fucking dishwater.

Year ten saw me unknowingly choosing economics as an elective then turning up for my first class with a kitchen apron. It hit me when I realised one of my best friends Matt, who was the school's equivalent to Steve Jobs, was in the class and I thought, *That's odd, he said his electives were introduction to maths methods, law and economics.* Then the penny dropped.

'Jackie, it's an economics class as in financial matters of the world, not home economics as in cooking! Wrong choice to say the least. You're not going anywhere though, so sit down, listen and learn.'

Well, it definitely got a laugh at least. I was in hell sitting through that class, as even the basics of budgeting of was never taught to me at home, let alone understanding the following:

- The S&P 500 is not about counting grains of salt and pepper equally.

- A Nasdaq is not the brand of a car in *Fast and Furious.*

- The stock exchange is in no way about people loaning each other ingredients for when they want to make soup.

- Bonds isn't just underwear.

Due to some sort of miracle, I was about to complete year ten. On a beautiful, sunny morning break in October, from a short distance away we could see one of our old class teachers, Mrs Caving, on duty. I decided to have a chat with her for the sake of just being annoying, as I was good at that. She was quite upper crust in her stance, and extremely noble in her pronunciation, just ripe for the picking in my mind. Clair asked her if the teachers had decided on what class we would be moving into once year eleven commenced. Out of the six girls waiting for her response, everyone got told their future teacher except one. Me. She stared down her finely chiselled nose and in a tone that could be heard fifty metres away said, 'Jackie, due to your grades this year we decided as a caring committed body of teachers to keep you down, therefore you will be repeating year ten.'

My world stopped. The blood drained from my body and all I could think was, *Holy shit, fuck, fuck, fuck!* I was in deep, deep trouble with my parents.

'Oh my God, you're kidding me?'

'I beg your pardon, young lady, do not use the Lord's name in vain.'

No that's right, I thought, *do it while I'm down*.

Quite frankly it couldn't get any worse at that stage. Whatever happened to pulling me aside gently and explaining my situation away from any prying ears so I didn't feel like a loner or different from the other kids? Oh, that's right; things were different in 1984. 'Just chuck her in the deep end, she'll either swim or sink.' I was definitely sinking fast.

I think she felt sorry for me. I begged her not to be so caring and just let me go up to year eleven in a herd with the rest of the flock. We were raised like sheep and I, all of a sudden, was going to be the only lamb to the slaughter. I even asked her to tell the other teachers to ignore me, that I wouldn't bother anyone. She didn't realise what circumstances she'd just unleashed, nor was she respondent to any of my suggestions.

Now was the time I needed to make my way to the tiny garden chapel up the back of school and get on my knees and pray. Pray very, very hard. I wasn't praying for forgiveness at my lack of trying to excel at school. I merely prayed for mercy and protection for when I was to return home that afternoon from school.

I don't know if you've ever experienced when you have bad news to share with someone and you don't know how you're going break it to them. I have a memory like an elephant but for the life of me I cannot recall what I was thinking from the time I prayed for the Lord's protection and guidance to the point of breaking the news to my parents. It's a total blank. I remember waiting for Dad to get home that afternoon so I could tell them at the same time so the wrath I knew I was going to endure was going to hit me all at once, probably quite literally. I prepared for a physical onslaught and I felt it a much better option that way than for it to be dragged out. That plan didn't eventuate though, did it?

Mum told me that we were going to be having a special treat together for dinner that night as Dad was at some charity function so he would not be home until way past my bedtime. What Mum failed to understand was that if I didn't get off my chest that which was also spinning around in my head I was going to implode.

There I was, in the kitchen after dinner with Mum, trying to look like I was enjoying 'girly time', as my brother was also out. Then she did it. She started looking really motherly at me for the first time in I couldn't recall how long and then it kicked in; her female, bloody motherly instinct.

'Sweetie, you look worried. What's on your mind? Go on. You can tell me ... I know that your father and I have been a bit hard on you lately, but we love you and—'

Blah, blah, blah.

My internal dialogue was asking her, *Why? Why are you concerned now? I mean, tonight, of all nights ... seriously, why? You've got to be fucking kidding me. What is wrong with people?*

I then launched into what can only be described as dysentery of the mouth, knowing full well she was going to lose it. The worst bit was Dad hadn't arrived home yet, so after telling her I was going to have to repeat it to him. I breathed deeply ... exhaled ... then spoke.

'Mrs Caving told me today I'll be repeating year ten.'

Then all I heard was white noise.

... Then it hit.

BANG!

The neighbours heard it – my mum, not the white noise. She turned from Mary Poppins into Cruella de Ville at record speed. She did the banshee thing she did back in 1981 again but with cardboard Riesling running through her blood stream. It was incredibly scary. I braced myself to be hit. Instead I got an onslaught of verbal rage, which makes me shudder today, even mentally recalling it. Then she said that thing every child dreads.

'When your father gets home ...'

Not bloody ten minutes after telling her, who should come through the front door but none other than Dad. Bloody hell, his timing was pathetic. Or was it mine?

She told him in no uncertain terms. No embellishment, just facts. That white noise again, it was quite deafening. Again, I braced for the hit. I wasn't disappointed this time. He knocked me to the ground, violently launching himself at me, shoving me over with both hands on my shoulders.

'You fucking hopeless little bitch.'

There was rage on his face, but he was wearing a suit and tie. It sounds odd but my thoughts immediately went to my belief that a man in a suit and a tie is a business man, a professional man, a gentleman.

My mother was yelling at him to stop. She pulled him away with everything she had.

'RUN! Go to your room. GO!'

I backed away, not having yet stood up. I was still in shock but at the same time I felt deserving of his physical blow. I crawled away on my hands, facing him until I felt safe enough to have him at my back where I couldn't see the rage on his face. I made it to my room then slammed the door. I slid my body down the wall until I was sitting on the floor with my back against my bedroom door in case he tried to open it. I obviously had high hopes that my frame could stop him entering my room. I slept by the door that night. The alcohol-fuelled screaming that went on was surely heard by our neighbours. No one complained though.

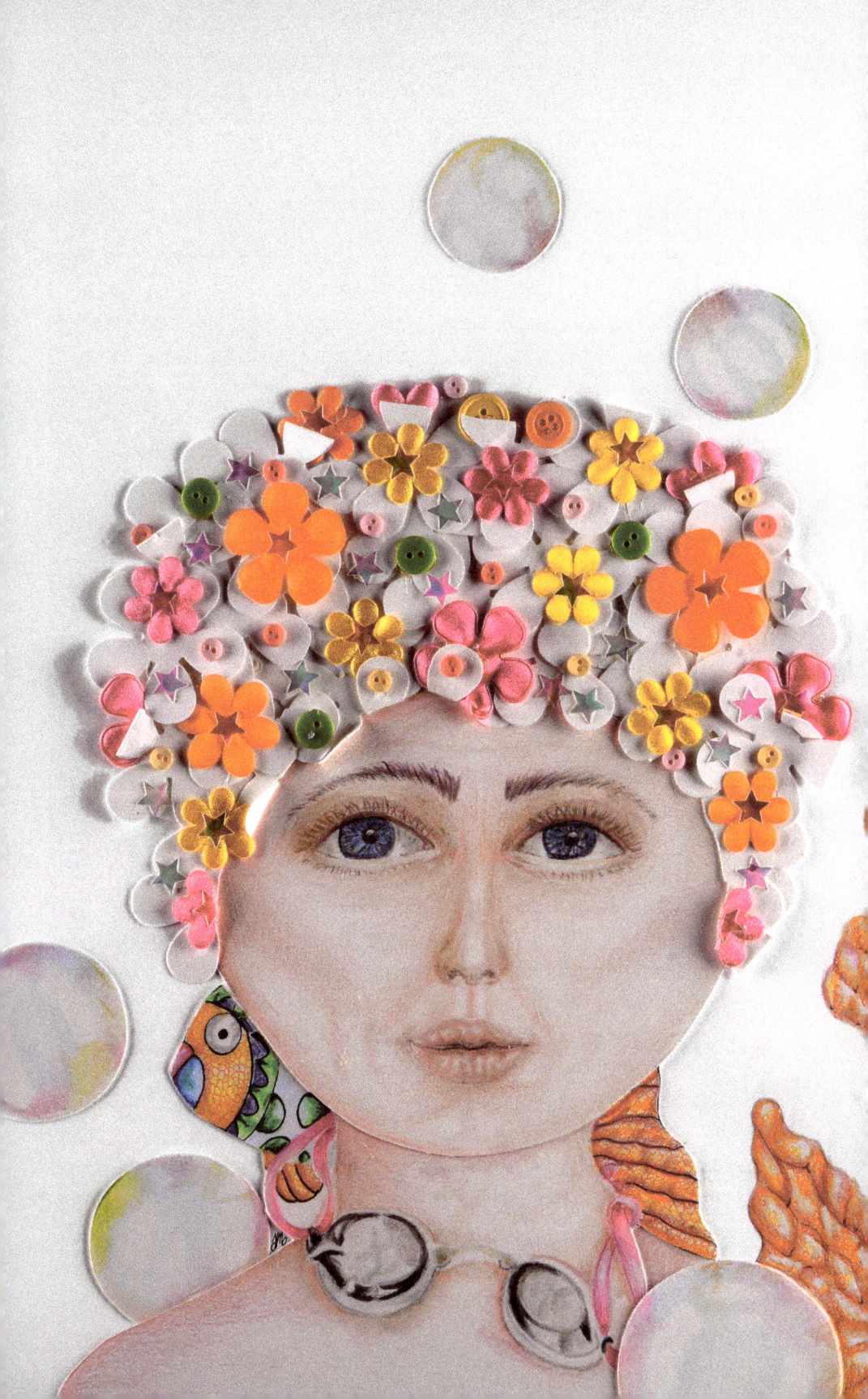

1985

I was returned to school after my failed attempt the previous year. My parents also threatened me with being sent back to the local public school again, but they sustained I'm sure it was only from the fact that it reflected badly on them from a social perspective. There's nothing like good old-fashioned embarrassment. So instead, they verbally subjected me to every name under the sun when they'd had too much to drink. Just a normal night, really. It was also highly recommended that I 'lay low' and keep out of their way. Something took place, though, that was to change the game plan.

I thought starting back at school that year would be difficult as I was repeating year ten, but my friends who went on to year eleven never left my side and I made friends in my new classes. I even started dating my first real boyfriend, Matt, in November of the previous year. We were a true juxtaposition; he was brilliant and I was, as my parents put it, brilliant at being stupid. We had been best friends since we were fourteen so it was comforting that I hadn't been left behind.

Arriving home from school one afternoon in 1985, I recall dropping my bag once through the door and walking over to raid the pantry. All of a sudden, I felt this sharp pain shoot up the back of my left thigh, to a point where I fell to the floor. The feeling then ran its way up to my lower back, to my coccyx.

'Jack, stop being a bloody drama queen,' Mum said.

I didn't know what was happening. I called out for help as I couldn't move. Mum finally realised I was truly in pain when I started crying so she decided to help me to my feet. When I stood, I was unable to walk properly. Placing my left heel on the ground caused a pain that would dig deeply into the back of my upper thigh. My analogy was that if I were a puppet, it was as though the string that controlled my left leg had been shortened. I couldn't put my left foot flat on the ground and walk properly as the pain was excruciating. The fun started when my eldest sister Anne, a nurse at the time, was told to get home and talk with me, as Mum didn't know what to do.

'Yes, she says she's in pain and can't put her foot down. I have no idea what to do. She's given your father and I so much trouble. You deal with her.'

Anne wholeheartedly took on the job of finding solutions to my health dilemma. That didn't just include the old school medical fraternity either. Over the next five months, I was sent to doctors, physiotherapists, paediatric psychologists, osteopaths and naturopaths.

True to form though, I never spoke a word about anything that was going on within the walls of our home, not even to my sisters, as it was considered irrelevant. I was constantly told I was being dramatic and to shut up – whatever happened, I felt insignificant and pointless. Why would anyone care? I didn't feel like a victim, I just didn't matter or want to cause a scene. Subconsciously, I never wanted to do anything to upset Dad. I was very protective of Mum and knew she'd be upset with me if I ever mentioned anything that reflected poorly on us as a family. I was raised to believe what went on under our family roof was normal. We were the 'perfect family', just as Mum said we were. We functioned on a level of perfection, every day, and that was that.

Through guidance of the physio, I was in an Olympic-size swimming pool every night doing laps for an hour. Even though I had developed great arm muscles and good core strength, the pain was only slightly relieved once in the water. When out of the pool I was extremely tired and when in school had a habit of falling asleep in class.

Chiropractors were visited and, no matter how soft they tried to be, when they manipulated my bones the pain was enormous, so every session ended in tears. I would get home exhausted, and miss the next morning's schooling, as I had to sleep it off. I was then given a full torso, thick woollen wrap back-brace with flat metal rods to wear. It sat under my school uniform to help support me but it had a down side. I was a sixteen-year-old girl who didn't walk like normal kids – you know, that cool swagger they have. I tended to attract attention. My personalised swagger looked as if I was trying to balance books on my head.

Our family doctor had come to a dead end on how to proceed with my back, so the next step was to see a surgeon. They'd realised it wasn't in my head, or something my body would fix by itself. In fact, it was getting worse.

In June, Mum and I made our way into East Melbourne to a surgeon named Mr Ray. He spent maybe half an hour watching me move in different ways. Then, after sending me to the Alfred Hospital for an MRI scan, a date was set to have a procedure where dye was injected into my spinal cord while I was under anaesthetic, so he could see where the nerves of my spine were hindering me.

As procedures go it was ground breaking but, unfortunately, had a bad side effect. The good news was the dye showed Mr Ray where and what the problem was in my spine. The bad news was that once I woke from the anaesthetic, I had to keep completely horizontal for the following twenty-four hours. If I stood up the dye would move up through my spinal cord and into my brain, giving me a migraine that could last a few days and here laid the problem.

After the procedure I had to get home from hospital and therefore I had to travel in a car, hence at some point I was to have my body in a position that was vertical. Due to Newton's Theory, I was overcome by a migraine that laid me low for three days and only added to the pain I was feeling within my back itself. I was left bedridden and terribly ill.

After Mr Ray had read the results of the test, a date was set for me to go into the hospital for a surgical spinal procedure. He was feeling positive it would stop the pain once and for all.

Mum booked a family holiday and the three of us went up to Noosa for a few weeks prior to the surgery. I clearly recall it was the loveliest family holiday ever. My parents were on their best behaviour towards me. I felt loved, safe and comfortable; it was so special. I think they realised how serious spinal surgery was and if something were to go wrong the result would be dreadful.

But I was oblivious to the whole thing. I really had no idea what I was in for. It's true what they say about ignorance being bliss.

To me, ignorance was also safe.

1985 – July

I received well wishes from friends and family up until the morning I was to enter the hospital, Mercy Private in East Melbourne. With Mum by my side, I was over the pain and ready to be operated on.

Once I was admitted to a private room, I was happily content. My nurse told me that I could order anything off the menu, twenty-four hours a day. I was completely over the moon. Chocolate milkshakes in abundance! Not straight away though, as I was due to go into the operating theatre at 2 pm that afternoon, so my swimmer's appetite had to wait. As the time of the operation grew closer, Mr Ray entered my room and sat by my bed to kindly explain to me what was about to take place.

I'd be wheeled into the operating theatre, but I wouldn't be administered with an anaesthetic that would put me to sleep. Instead, I would need to stay awake for the procedure, but the anaesthetist was going to give me what was called an epidural. As a teenage girl I didn't have the faintest idea about childbirth, let alone what an epidural was. So, of course, this wasn't to be an issue to me. I was excitedly thinking, *Ok, let's do this thing and get it over with. I've got to get back to my room and order off the menu.*

That was until I was in the surgical theatre. The attending nurse and the anaesthetist were kind enough to show me the needle that was going to be injected into my spinal cord. Wrong move on their part. I believe the correct description of a horse tranquiliser would give you an idea of how big the needle was. I was told the whole procedure would take only half an hour and I would be returned, drinking chocolate milkshakes in no time. I should have requested it in writing.

Mr Ray asked me to lay on my left side with my knees as far up against my chest as I could manage. I squeezed up into a tight ball, which was hard as my leg restricted me greatly. Then he started to administer the drug via the enormous needle into the crack in my one of my vertebrae he had found in the dye procedure. It was to be placed directly through the crack into my spine. Unfortunately, it wasn't the textbook job he thought it would be.

He really did try his hardest to get the needle through the crack, and I mean he was quite forceful. I understand now why they put you to sleep during surgical procedures: it's so you don't get to witness how roughly they treat your body. Instead of the time quoted by Mr Ray, the needle probing went on for just over an hour and a half. It was my job to stay awake and listen to Mr Ray's instructions as to how to position my spine so the needle could be inserted into the correct place. I waited and waited. With the pain came adrenaline and then exhaustion. All I could hear was Mr Ray telling the nursing staff that he couldn't get the needle through the crack in my spine.

'It's OK, Jackie, hang in there ... it won't be long now ... are you OK?'

There was instruction after instruction.

'Can you pull your legs up tighter into your chin ... no, no, can't feel it ... can you feel anything? Wait, I think I've got it ... no, pulling out again. Nurse, I need a new needle.'

The needle had bent and the pain was so bad I felt I went into another headspace.

When I was finally returned to my room I was physically and emotionally spent. Before I fell asleep, Mum and Mr Ray came into my room to tell me that I would be returning to the operating theatre the following morning as there had been a problem: either that or he was a sadist. I was scheduled to undergo spinal surgery at eleven the next morning. He had found the problem to my past six months of agony. He described the events of administering the day's procedure to Mum.

'It was like trying to find a needle in a haystack, Mrs Ellwood.'

I wanted to tell him that from my perspective the story was that I felt like a voodoo doll being attacked by a disgruntled psychopath, but I refrained. Mr Ray via his needle probing had found a large crack in my lower vertebrae. When this crack occurred, he didn't know. Then it came to me. I knew. I knew when and how it had happened, but still didn't speak up.

What had physically occurred, though, was a nerve had settled and caught in my spine where the crack was, so when it was healing the nerve was crushed. That's why I was feeling the pain running down my left leg, making it difficult to walk.

I stared at my doctor; I was in an exhausted daze, thinking I needed the pain to stop. To this day I do not have a problem with needles because I feel nothing could be worse than what I experienced. I had officially become a human pincushion.

As to how the nerve had been caught in a crack in my spine, there were two stories. Both events took place but one of the stories, which I'll call the 'horse story', was used to cover up the other, true story of Dad kicking me in the back and breaking my coccyx. It was told not only to the medical fraternity but family and friends who always asked after the operation when my thick, ugly red scar was on show. It was like show and tell. Dad would say, 'Jack, show them your scar!' I'd lift up the back of my t-shirt and lower the back of my jeans. People would gasp at how grotesque it looked.

The truth of my broken back was never raised. It never was a topic of conversation between Dad and me ever. I found other ways of dealing with it, again to my detriment.

I recall my first encounter with the drug morphine and I will hold it closely to my heart because it sustained me and kept me company before and after my operation that was to take place on that sunny but cold July Melbourne morning. Once administered it never took long until I was warmly comforted without a care.

Entering the operating theatre, I was gently transferred onto the table, and then administered with a stint in my left hand by the anaesthetist. Mr Ray gently spoke to me, reminding me that today I was not going to remember a thing. The anaesthetist asked me kindly to start counting backwards from ten.

I got to seven then passed out.

After a six-hour operation, I was woken up.

'Jackie, honey, it's all over, sweetie! Jack, Jack, Jack!'

Oh Lord, stop repeating my name, it is echoing over and over and over.

I vomited.

I remember waking up in a room with just my bed. Mum was sitting by my side and I looked out my window. It was dusk.

'Where's Dad?'

I passed out again.

Where's Dad? Mum, where's Dad?

I kept dreaming about seeing him but he never came. The man who was responsible for what I had just been through and was now enduring was the only person I wanted to see the most. I didn't want to yell in rage about what his actions had caused. I wanted him to comfort me. Nothing came.

I didn't see him for another two weeks. I was told he was too busy to get away from work. The afternoon he did drop in, he was there for only a few minutes and a friend accompanied him. Mum had asked if there was anything Dad could bring in for me and I remember asking her if he could bring me in a little floral posse of violets from Keven O'Neil's florist in Toorak. I was very interested in floristry and he was the best in Australia. Dad had promised me flowers before I entered hospital. When he entered my room, I was so happy to see him. It was a confirmation that he hadn't forgotten about me. As he left I was feeling a bit cheeky, so I asked him where he was hiding the violets he had promised me.

He turned and said, 'Bugger off, Jack. You're not worth it.'

Much laughter ensued with his business colleague and then he was gone. I didn't see him again until I returned home weeks later.

One of my warmest memories of being holed up in hospital for that length of time was on 15 July 1985. I watched Bob Geldof's Live Aid concert on TV. I didn't have anything else to do so I watched the whole thing with a few new friends I'd met in there.

My favourite friend was a young girl called Penny who had her mouth wired and neck in a sturdy brace. She was unable to walk because she'd been in a car accident after her father had gotten behind the wheel of the family car after drinking with mates in their backyard. He'd told her she had to go to the bottle shop with him and buy his grog as he was too drunk and they wouldn't let him purchase anything in that state. Penny was sent flying through the car's front window, lucky to get away with her life. I thought it pathetic that going for your pen licence as an eight-year-old was harder than the opportunity of having children. He came out of it without a scratch – his alcohol-flooded body rolled with the motion of the out-of-control vehicle.

We watched a very young Madonna, Queen, Wham, Eurhythmics – the list went on and on. I laid flat next to Penny as her TV was bolted to the ceiling so she had some form of entertainment.

1986

I started working at a fur and leather boutique. If I knew at the time that a Mink was actually a cute, little, furry animal and not the name of a coat every wealthy woman in the 80s dreamed of owning, I would have happily thrown red paint over my boss and yelled profanities at him every day, as he was an arsehole. He illegally kept boxes of emu, crocodile and snake leather shoes in the attic of our shop for his wealthiest customers. They were unlawfully made for the guys at Melbourne's Stock Exchange in Collins Street. Nothing like a crocodile on each foot after a few lines of cocaine to make you feel like you're king of the road.

I was young and wanted to have some fun meeting other people, but there was one problem: I was green. All I wanted was for someone to ask me out on a date. Simple, right? They did eventually but my wish didn't go as I hoped.

I supposedly caught the eye of a tall and very handsome young guy who worked in sales for Pioneer on Swanston Street a few doors down from where I worked. His name was Ben and he invited me to lunch one day, only to tell me that he already had a girlfriend but wanted to introduce me to a mate of his. Odd, really, but I agreed. We went back to his workplace surrounded by sound systems and I was introduced to his boss, a very well-dressed bloke in his thirties. I felt immediately that I was punching above my weight as I'd only been out with Matt. Then the boss asked me out the back of the shop for a chat. I obliged. He informed me that he was married.

What the hell, what is it with these guys? I thought.

He then said he had a friend who he wanted to match me up with on a blind date. The plot thickened. Seriously, it was like a joke! How many men does it take to set Jackie up a date? Obviously, a truckload. I should have cut my losses and walked away then, but I stupidly didn't. He assured me this guy was single and a great bloke who needed a date for a party that was being arranged in his honour. All I heard was the word party. I thought, *Great, I get to buy a new dress and shoes.* I gave him my home number and told the manager I'd chat to his friend first before deciding on going out with him.

The mystery man called that night and I found out his name was Max. We chatted, and he sounded nice enough, so we agreed to meet down at my local train station on Saturday night. Mum would drop me off. I specifically remember Dad commenting about me going on my first date with an adult male.

'That's fine, but don't bring him here!'

So much for mixed message parental guidance.

Saturday night. I arrived in Mum's car at the station and first thing I noticed was that Max looked good. Second thing: he was very polite to my mother. If she wasn't happy with what she saw she would've stopped the date going ahead very quickly. And to round it all off he picked me up in a white Jaguar sports coupe XS. Name me one seventeen-year-old girl who wouldn't be excited to be going to an adult party with an older, hot-looking guy in a sports car ... thought not. OK, I take that back. If you were a responsible teenager and understood the 1980s decree of 'stranger danger' you wouldn't have contemplated it, but responsibility was not a part of my vocabulary. I didn't even know how to spell it.

We drove to Max's place first as he informed me these types of parties don't start until about 11 pm. He knew that my curfew was 12.30 am, so I was wondering how it was going to work.

Once inside his home in Templestowe, which was a three-storey split-level, I could see it was very well decorated, for the late 1980s anyway. There was white leather décor with polished large white tiles, peachy hues and potted palm trees everywhere. Very chic.

I sat. We made small talk while he poured a drink. I found out that he was a professional freelance fashion photographer whose work appeared in *Harper's Bazaar* and *Vogue* magazines. He was obviously well travelled, and had photographed my idol Jerry Hall, the one and only true supermodel of the 80s, in my opinion. I was so excited to see the signed photo on his desk of the two of them on a beach in St Barts. It read, *Darling*

Max, you're the best. Love, Jerry oxoxo. Apart from all the added materialistic bonuses a seventeen-year-old thinks of, I realised he seemed like a nice guy.

Max then informed me that he didn't really want to go to the party, as his divorce had just come through from his wife. His friends were holding the party in his honour to welcome him back into the single life he once led. After I finished my drink, he asked me if I smoked.

I answered edgily. 'I sure do, been smoking since I was thirteen, up the back of my school.'

I felt extremely grown up, especially since my parents had allowed me to start drinking at sixteen, as well as going to night cubs. I was born with a Benson & Hedges in my mouth. After going through gestation with Mum smoking a packet and a half a day, I was committed to the cause ... and the effects.

Max replied, 'Ah, no Jackie,' with a smug look on his face. 'I mean weed.'

With a stupid smile plastered on my face, in a high-pitched voice I answered, 'Oh, that ... sure.'

I'm very sure he could tell I was lying to cover up being so unsophisticated. I had never touched drugs in my life and in 1986 neither alcohol nor cigarettes were considered drugs.

It was that night at Max's that I tried weed for the first time. I had my first and last bong. It's a horrid-looking apparatus, so ill-designed, with no aesthetic potential in it whatsoever. Weed did nothing for me, and thank goodness for that.

After a few drinks I asked Max when we were going to the party. He dropped a bomb.

'Jackie, I really like your company, and I'd much prefer to stay here until I have to drive you home.'

I didn't understand; I was gutted. Did he think I was a child?

Obviously noticing my distress, Max then explained it to me. 'The party that is being put on for me tonight is a swinger's party.'

'What's that?' I asked. 'I can dance you know.'

'No.' He was highly amused at my answer. 'We would drive to a friend's home, and there would be about thirty couples there. There's a strong possibility that the men that will be there will ask you to go into one of the bedrooms with them and have sex, maybe even a married couple together.'

I was staring at him with my mouth open and brows raised, trying to comprehend what he was telling me.

'Sorry, I don't understand.'

He continued. 'But it is consensual, so if you didn't want to, you wouldn't have to!'

What Max didn't realise was that I had a major problem saying no to anyone. It was not because I neither wanted everything nor was difficult to please. It was the fact that I never wanted to upset anyone. Therefore, I hardly ever said no and it was always to my detriment. No was a word that I was never allowed to use at home; it was always yes. Yes, Dad. Yes, Mum. I was not taught how to argue a point or think for myself (or so I believed). I'm sure I could have been the poster girl for American therapist and emotional abuse expert Beverly Engel when she wrote the book *The Nice Girl Syndrome*. That was me for a very long time. It's not only exhausting but opens you up to mistreatment by others on an epic scale. When raised by a father who drinks and who has a fanciful mindset to trust everyone due to an intoxicated, overreaching optimism, and who says time and again he knows better than you, you are destined to fail. There is no safeguard you can hold onto, only the belief that if you treat everyone honestly then they will surely reciprocate. If you live in a decent society, that might happen but there will come a time where it won't and you will fail dismally, becoming a victim to abuse in its many forms.

I was six when Dad put me in the cabin of a truck that had arrived at our home to pick up rubbish he was clearing from our garage. The driver, a complete stranger, didn't know how to get to the rubbish tip that was a fifteen-minute drive away.

'Here, take my daughter Jack. She'll show you where it is,' Dad said.

I remember feeling so scared, kneeling on the seat so I could see out the window, thinking that if I stayed quiet, he wouldn't notice me sitting there. An hour later I was returned home. Dad was angry. Angry that his six-year-old daughter didn't know where she was going. Mum was upset that I'd upset Dad.

In life I'd developed into a kitten with a ball of wool; everything was playful. I was so very grateful that there and then Max made a decision on my behalf. It was obvious to him I was not the type of person who was mature enough to be taken to such an event. He returned me home by my curfew time and, even though we went out to dinner the following evening, I never saw him again after that.

I was still to remain green for quite a while after that too.

Life started to lose its innocence that day. I was living a naïve existence and I was going to have to toughen up very quickly if I were to keep my sanity. Unfortunately, I didn't learn quickly enough.

1988

Our family business was in retail but it was something I never envisioned a career in. I needed something other than just customer service. I needed to prove to myself that I could meet challenges in something I was proud to do.

I found the courage to apply for a place at RMIT to study visual merchandising including fine arts and photography in Melbourne's CBD. I was ecstatic to be accepted and for the first time I really felt a sense of belonging and achievement.

The following year I started classes. One afternoon when I left my last class of the day, later than normal, something occurred that changed my life and sent me on a destructive path I could never have imagined.

Normally I would walk to Flagstaff station with one of my classmates, Dale. Unfortunately, on this day I didn't, as I had to stay back to finish a photography project because the darkroom was free. At around 4.30 I was making my way up the laneway that gave students easy access to the train station. Even though it was normally bustling with people, on this cool but sunny autumn afternoon it was vacant. No one was in sight. As I got a third of the way up the lane, I noticed four men. They would have been in their mid-thirties, walking down on the opposite side of the road towards me. A few seconds later, they all moved onto my side of the lane. Around that time there was a lot of new development going on in the legal district of Melbourne and there was scaffolding and solid fencing up so passers-by couldn't go anywhere near the construction site. As I was getting further up the hill these guys were getting nearer. I could tell by the language they were speaking that they were of a European background. I recall thinking that, as I had on a solid backpack and was holding a large A1 size folio, I was to keep to the left so naturally these guys would move as we got closer. That didn't happen.

As they were talking and laughing between themselves, they walked right up to me in unison, creating a human wall of sorts. I immediately and naively thought, *They're busy chatting and haven't noticed me. They're not going to move. I will.* I immediately diverted to my right, which put me in the middle of the group. I had nowhere else to go. Suddenly, I was picked up by a large hand holding the crotch of my jeans, another hand on my shoulder. He lifted me up then slammed me into a solid ply building wall, winding me. I don't know who did what but a hand was put over my mouth while another hand went up my shirt onto my breast. It was squeezed so hard it later formed a huge bruise. Another hand was shoved down the front of my pants, making its way into my underpants to fondle me. Rough callused fingers were thrust inside me, hard nails scraping inside my vagina. The dank smell of liquor on their breath and cigarette-stained hands on my mouth I can still recall today and a version of myself, pathetically mustering up a scared and muffled cry that no one could hear.

It all happened so quickly but felt like forever before it stopped. Next thing I knew, I was on the ground. They had just dropped me, like a limp doll, casually walking off, laughing down the road again like nothing happened. One of them turned back to look at me, calling out a word I hadn't heard before.

'Puttana!' He then spat on the ground.

I went blank.

Shakily, I finally got on my feet, tried to tuck my shirt into my pants and collected my bag and folio. With tears flowing down my face, I frantically ran to the station looking for the police but saw none. On the train home the image of what had just occurred to me played over and over again in my mind. I kept checking my clothing to make sure I was covered up, to not show any signs of what had just happened. I couldn't work out in my head what I'd done to deserve it.

Where did I go wrong? What did I do wrong? Think. Think! What did I do?

Time and again I clenched my pelvic floor muscles trying to clear away the feeling inside myself, a remnant of his deep grazing. I was desperate to get home. When I arrived, I was not greeted with the support I so desperately needed. Running down the driveway to the door, I hurriedly reached for the handle but couldn't get in as it was locked. Mum obviously noticed my stress so came and opened the door. As soon as she did, I burst into tears and my mind and body went into shutdown. She then grabbed and shook me, trying to work out what was wrong. I couldn't speak; I just couldn't put into words what had occurred. Her reaction was to do only as she thought appropriate; she swung her open hand as hard as she could muster, slapping my face. She left a mark on my already aching body, but this mark was to show on my cheek.

I was in complete shock. I was finally able to stop hyperventilating long enough to ask why she did it.

She yelled at me. 'What the hell is the matter with you? Stop it!'

In between trying to tell her what had happened and trying to steady my quivering voice, I told her the shortened version – that a couple of guys grabbed me in the city on the way home.

'For God's sake, go and wash your face. Your father will be home soon ... and don't mention it to him as he's had a bad day.'

And that was all that was ever said.

Instead of washing my face, I got into a hot shower. I couldn't warm up. I scrubbed myself all over with a nailbrush, even my genital area, still unable to get clean. There was fresh red blood on my underwear from a scratch inside my vagina. I unconsciously put the thought of it away in my brain within the heavily guarded box marked: Warning! Do Not Open. I didn't want to cause any trouble and in a split second decided to live with it. I wasn't prepared go anywhere near the issue until nearly twenty-three years later. My coping strategy was to think that I must have done something to deserve it.

But that box had a lot of shameful experiences shoved into it already, to a point where it could not hold its shape for much longer. Something was going to happen that would eventually trigger its implosion. And the reason I say implosion is because you are the only one who feels the damage that has been done to you over time. You are the one collapsing from the weight of a mix of muffled emotions, guilt, anger, frustration and rage.

From being bent out of shape in so many ways through my father's abuse and now sexual assault from male strangers, I was put under immense pressure without the recourses to explain my demise or breakdown. It was the tipping point of feeling like I couldn't cope any longer. Coping alone isn't a healthy tool unless you're eventually able to meet your problems head on. Coping isn't living; coping is existing within the turmoil of your own mind. I had not a sliver of an idea of how to, so I gave up without a fight. Everything I cared about and loved came falling down even though this event was not to be the undoing of me because, like the little trooper I was raised to be, I put on a mask again and continued along a visionless path. An empty hollow path. Self-loathing hit a new high.

1989

Not long after the attack, some of my closest relationships started to disintegrate. This was when my partying and spending went up to a new level. I splurged on anyone who came into my space. My drinking was becoming a problem behind closed doors, as I just couldn't muster up the courage to face another day at times. I'd have breakfast before getting on the train for the city but I'd be consuming a Patra orange juice spiked heavily with gin, arriving to class feeling composed and nonchalant. Once morning class had ended, I'd be rolling up to The Golden Age pub on King Street with my classmates in tow to spend an afternoon playing pool and drowning a few more beers. Strangely enough though, my grades were reaping high distinctions from me filtering my anger and grief into my art, no matter the medium. I couldn't speak about it so I put it into different outlets of art. I tried to hit a nerve with anyone who chose to notice.

It was 1989 and I had to dress a window on King Street in Melbourne for a Mother's Day campaign that was being graded. Whilst under the influence, I decided to dress my mannequins, which I placed in provocative positions, in black and red lace underwear, including garter belts and stockings and the highest black patent leather heels I could find. I sunk over two hundred dollars into it, which was a lot of money back then. And it paid in spades. The window read: Be Risqué This Mother's Day. Before the day was over, I was pulled out of class by the principal. There had been a car accident out front of the school and my window was being blamed for it. It was the first time I really stood up for myself. I was hungover and angry. It was just another day, really.

'Are you kidding me? I was given a brief and I met it. I was graded on it and I received better marks than anyone else did. You marked it, Stephen.'

I was stabbing the air, pointing at my lecturer.

I continued. 'My job is to make people notice a product and I did that. If some dickhead gets hard and runs into another car because of my art, that's his problem, not mine.'

Then I started ugly crying – the crying I did when I didn't get my way. Calm dialogue was something I'd yet to master and it would take many more years to understand that it was the best path to take when communicating as an adult. I did everything but stamp my feet.

'You call us artists. That's what you're meant to nurture and support, not berate me for doing my job, for expressing myself. You wouldn't have pulled one of the guys up for this. You've got an issue that it has to do with sex and I'm a woman. It's bullshit.'

There was no evidence at all of that but I felt victimised and I was angry. Deep down I was glad it upset them. I wanted a fight.

'Jackie, please calm down. We've not had a window like this before and on review it might have crossed the line.' Stephen was calm and could see how upset I was. 'I promise you your mark won't change but we can't keep the installation. It'll have to come down immediately.'

Now I was fuming. 'Then you two take the fucking thing down. I'm going to the pub. And whatever you do, don't ruin my merchandise, I need to return it and get my money back. You're all fucking gutless.'

I stormed out, slamming the door and headed to my favourite place, a dark table that sat on sticky carpet that smelled of a mixture of beer and cigarettes. My second home, The Golden Age. Nursing a Corona, I resorted to crying. Thank God I had a few classmates join me to commiserate. They consoled me and bought me drinks. I was so enraged and it only antagonised my already battered ego. I knew I'd crossed the line, but I wanted to push boundaries, in many areas of my life, including in my relationships.

I'd been dating a guy called Preston for a few years and we had a wonderful time together. He was such a decent person and I felt very lucky to call him my boyfriend. He was a very respectful, highly intelligent, funny guy and to top it off he had a brilliant relationship with his parents and siblings. I really enjoyed being a part of his family as it was the complete opposite of what I had experienced in my own. But after the attack, the goings-on of what is considered a so-called normal relationship became a strain in my mind. Sex had to be rougher and harder. I had this enormous urge to be hit and to be abused. I started to behave terribly, pushing him away, but he still stayed by my side. I went from a young woman with so much to seeing everything as wrong, nothing was good enough, I felt I deserved better – I was entitled.

Preston knew I'd been attacked but not to what extent. I never told him out of fear it was my fault. He booked me into self-defence classes so I could protect myself. He even spent nights with me in my parent's rumpus room, practising protecting myself, but no amount of learning how to knee a bloke in the balls was going to help me. It had left its irreversible mark. The paranoia was the worst bit – waiting to be approached by men, seeing them out of the corner of my eye, thinking that I was being followed. I'm sure he thought I was going crazy, being overly dramatic. I was so scared and confused. I had reason to be overwhelmed but my mother refused to acknowledge it and my sisters were never told. I wasn't allowed to bring it up, so it stayed buried.

I deliberately started pushing people away. Deep down I'd like to think I asked myself why I needed help but just couldn't verbalise why, but in truth maybe I never really tried. To be angry was easier, to pick a fight was easier, to cause a drama-fuelled incident that would rile everyone else up was easier. It was easier than to sit with a feeling that would mean I'd be left submerged in complete paranoia, my mind repeating the violation on auto-play.

My spending became more prevalent too. It felt so good to pay for possessions with money I'd skimmed from the pile of cash my father had given me the previous night. It never entered my mind that I was being abused or violated but I knew that what I had been experiencing as a person was wrong, so someone had to pay for it. It was my job to sort his businesses banking for the girls at his local branch. I was working two jobs while at uni but spending his money was more satisfying. The days takings, which I'd sort into upright denominations, were then given to the bank girls he'd flirt with, the girls he'd pick flowers for from our garden, the girls he'd buy jewellery for as gifts. Once Mum found out though, he'd have to buy a better trinket for her, and he'd always feel guilty when drunk and tell her. It was completely insane. I'd hear the yelling behind their bedroom door in all hours of the night because he was fucking her over too, and she stayed like a loyal dog. It made me ill.

One night I was heading out to dinner with Dad and Mum and I couldn't help myself. 'What's that smell? It's sickening.'

'Oh, your father bought it for me. It's Estée Lauder, Youth Dew. You don't like it? He says it reminds him of Cheryl from the bank,' Mum said shyly.

Putting my fingers on my temple and hanging my head in disbelief, all I could think was, *Oh my God, you are pathetic.*

I was an empty young woman who on the inside had no self-worth at all. I was hollow but from the outside I looked composed and in control. I was on track to a great career in art and fashion, but towards others I couldn't stop making openly snide remarks at their expense to a point where I knew I was getting a reputation of having an acid tongue. I was not funny, just nasty, and if you were at the end of my so-called quick wit, my words would hit you hard. I'd be invited to parties because I was fun to be around but, once there, I would drink to a point of being asked to leave due to trying to pick fights with other guests or passing out.

It was a miracle my body didn't shut down from what I was putting in it. If I went out clubbing, I'd start the night by putting away any alcohol I could get my hands on. My favourite was a shot mix of gin, vodka, vermouth and tequila. I'd become so infuriated for no reason at times and I just let the feeling stream through me. Everyone else had the problem. My ethos had become 'to eat or be eaten', which was so against my true nature, but something had changed. I had turned into a gutless bully, and I wholeheartedly loathed myself. Textbook passive aggression.

When we both turned twenty-three, Preston asked me to move into a flat with him. We bought a dog and all seemed fine from the outside, but not inside my head. Living with me must have been hell. Our relationship only lasted a year after that.

On a cold spring morning, after I had just walked in the front door after spending two weeks in Mitcham Private Hospital with alcohol-induced pancreatic inflammation, Preston decided to tell me our seven-year relationship was over. On the inside I knew it was nearing because I pushed the boundaries until they fell over a cliff. Packing my car, all I could think about was how grateful I was he'd finally broken it off. It started seven years prior. Something so special now in the gutter.

Behind the scenes I was devastated. I adored him but my attitude was inexcusable. He was such a decent person. For all the bitching, whining and abhorrent behaviour he put up with he probably no longer recognised the sweet girl he started dating years prior. I had become a nightmare.

I had an amazing job after finishing uni with a nationwide visual merchandising company. I worked alongside a prestigious team of creative individuals who spent eleven months of the year making then installing the Myer Christmas windows in the Bourke Street Mall in Melbourne. That was until the day I became so hyper-manic and anxious for no apparent reason.

I was driving my boss' car to collect some parts that were required. I was on the road and then the next minute my adrenalin level hit one hundred. I had no way of explaining what happened as I started taking huge risks behind the wheel, swerving in and out of traffic. I passed a stationary vehicle that was turning right on the outside but, as I swerved, I took a side mirror out of a parked car to my left. Once I returned to our workshop, I took the turn for the driveway at a speed too high then sped into the car park. I scraped all the side panels of the vehicle up against a brick wall. It was the right side and I was so close to the wall that I had to exit via the passenger door. My heart raced incredibly fast like I'd never experienced before.

The seriousness of what had happened didn't register and I just walked back into the factory and threw the keys on his desk. Not long after, my boss, Ron, headed out to his car to go to lunch and saw the damage. Within the hour I was politely called into his office and told I would be made redundant so it didn't blemish my job record. I was a good worker but at times my erratic behaviour had become impossible to predict, and it was occurring way too often.

Another visual merchandising job followed for a major jewellery company, which consisted of travelling all over the state. My weight had dropped terribly as I was living by myself and not eating. I had too much energy to eat, so I'd end up in bed sick quite often with colds turning into bronchitis. I'd endured a morning of being accosted by the boss' trophy wife when I'd finally had enough. She was asking me why I had the last two days off work, and saying if I wasn't looking after my health, she would have to speak to me formally via the Human Resources Department. I quit on the spot, thinking, *Fuck you both*. To top off my day, without giving it a second thought, I went and treated myself to a self-designed tattoo. There wasn't one sign of stability in my life; there was only the rush of what was next.

Finding work was my speciality but keeping it was another matter. I had the pretentious ability to see gaining a job as a fusion of confidence and delusion, the perspective of 'Try me, I'll land any job' and 'If I don't like it once I get it, I'll leave, get another anyway'. It was that simple and if you couldn't see it that was because you were holding yourself back – anyone could do it. When I was manic jobs were like a library of assignments. I sampled jobs like an open buffet. I was unstoppable but, obviously, it's not stable. Once I had a job an employer would offer a first day to see how things panned out. It was common, as I'd gain work by just walking off the street into the business that took my fancy. I'd work that first day and get paid cash for it then when asked if I'd like to join the team I'd say, 'No, thank you. It's not really for me'. I'd walk and do it again the following day. I became inebriated on the speed at which I could gain others' approval. Once I'd gained it, though, it was worthless to me.

Our family's business had a revolving door for my sake. I was in a true victim state of mind and hated going back to work with Dad but I felt I had no other option at times; I truly couldn't see any other way. When I was high, I could achieve anything. When it wore off and I couldn't get out of bed, he rode in on his mighty steed, berating my unhinged capacity to live a chaotic life and picking up the pieces. He loved it. I was hopeless and he was the saviour.

I seemed to stuff up everything that was placed in front of me. Looking back, I was handed so much on a platter, but I passionately tossed it all away. I could say I had a spoilt youth but the damage, the risks I took and my behaviour wasn't typical; I was unstable but was considered talented and artistic.

To be considered ill was never plausible. A dear friend once said to me in passing, 'Jack, you're eccentric and so much fun. You're intense. Truly, have you ever thought of being a comedian?' Then immediately flipped to the other side. 'In saying that, though, you can also suck the energy out of people, and you're demanding on others' time but I'm not sure you realise it. Shit, you're the whole package!' That was me to a tee.

Working for Dad had become a laughing matter for all his employees too. Why I was always returning to someone who treated me so poorly was something that would take me a long time to learn. As a small child I remember waking up in the middle of the night and becoming excited about working alongside him in the family business and how I could make it even more of a success than he had. I thought that would impress him but what I failed to understand time and again was he never did like being upstaged – ever. Every idea I came up with he returned serve with a negative comment.

To top it off also I wasn't a boy – I wasn't his son. I was his daughter. I was a girl and girls couldn't do anything in his mind, they were too weak, irrelevant. I was starved of his affection and I was willing to put up with whatever he dished out; I still needed his acknowledgment, his acceptance. Unconditional love was never on offer from Dad and yet I couldn't cope without him.

It wasn't long after my breakup from Preston when I distinctly recall saying to myself angrily that the next person I dated was going to treat me like a queen. Unfortunately, though, I'd forgotten I had to go out into public in order to meet new people. I tried to enjoy the process of meeting guys but it wasn't going to be that easy – I was still too angry.

1995

One-night stands were not my thing, never had been.

I decided I'd like to date again, but he would have to be the type of guy who would do anything for me. He would be not only decent and a gentleman, but he had to be worthy of me. I wouldn't date just anyone; I didn't have the patience or the time. I had an enormous ego-driven checklist and I wanted the best partner possible to give me everything on it – emphasis on give. But you should always be careful what you ask for, as you just might get it.

No one had explained, and I wouldn't have listened anyway because I thought I knew everything, how to appreciate anything, so it's only natural that I threw it all away, and with spectacular gusto.

His name was Charles. Charlie came from a very wealthy Melbourne family and promised me the world. He called me his princess – I wasn't a queen yet but it was close enough. After twelve months of dating, he proposed and we started looking for a house to buy. Our search took us to a new development in Kew. We drove to the site, about 7 kilometres from Melbourne's CBD and, as we parked, I could see a beautiful historic building that stood proudly on the north-facing hill. Once inside the plans were laid out in front of us and people were excitedly buzzing around looking at display rooms as the actual homes were yet to be built. There was commotion around some of the smaller rooms on show. The estate agent informed us they were smaller apartments available for purchase.

'They were the original asylum apartments that have been converted.'

'I'm sorry. What do you mean by asylum apartments?'

He spoke like a fully informed salesman, proud of his knowledge.

'The historic building you see on the hill was the Kew Asylum. It has surrounding cottages. It's where they housed the mentally

ill from 1887 and it was actually once known as the Kew Idiot Asylum. But this is prime land now and these apartments and houses are selling fast. You'll be buying a piece of Melbourne's history, and it will hold its value.'

It hit me quickly and I felt physically sick.

'So the insane lived here. People died here.' It was all I could think about.

'Well, yes, but people die every day, everywhere. It's not a cemetery, if that's what you're thinking.' He was sounding cocky now, like my statement was foolish.

Charlie could see through my facade and I was starting to look very unimpressed. 'Can you give us a minute?'

The estate agent walked away towards another interested party.

'Jack, what is it? This is a really good buy for something so close to the city,' Charlie asked me.

'Charlie, something happened here, I can feel it. It isn't right. This is the site of a mental asylum. You just can't go and build a house on land that may have housed and treated people who were seen as mentally insane and called idiots. I can only imagine what went on here but it feels very wrong. I can't stay here.'

I walked off to the car. Charlie followed, obviously thinking we'd missed out on the biggest real estate coup in years. We drove home in silence.

I couldn't convey how I felt that day. It was as if something was telling me I wasn't welcome on that site, that it was bad, it was rancid. In the past I'd driven along Princess Street time and again looking up at the building admiring the architecture, but ignorant to its history. Standing on its grounds was very different.

I was only to learn eight years later that my great-grandmother was admitted to Reception House at Kew on 31 December 1913. Mary was seventy-three at the time. She had been diagnosed as insane. She died, still in the Kew Asylum hospital, a little over seven months later, on 30 July 1914. The full extent of the coronial inquest I wasn't to learn until some twenty-six years later.

From my perspective, living there was never an option. It was then I knew why.

Charlie and I finally found a house further out of town and this one felt right. We settled in pretty quickly and, even though we were planning a wedding, my father had a light bulb moment. As per normal, all I wanted to do was please him.

My parents decided to sell their successful business that they'd had for forty-five years. They thought it would be wonderful for me to take it over with Charlie's help, so his father was brought in to financially back us. Looking back, it wasn't really a good reason to buy a business but whatever made our parents happy Charlie was happy to deliver on and, true to form, he did. I was able to keep a few of Dad's staff so we started over with a small but excited team. One of the new staff members was my best friend Scarlett, who I'd met at another company where I was a state visual mechanising trainer.

I worked during the day as a supervisor for a telecommunications company. At night I would visually merchandise the shop and organise the buying of stock. I still felt terribly unhappy. Back then depression just wasn't spoken about, not in my family anyway. I recall trying to explain it to Mum one day as my wedding dress was being fitted. She had worked so hard on choosing the material and organising everything – I just didn't have the patience to organise anything with working two jobs. She hit the roof.

'Jack, just get yourself together, *no one cares*. I have done everything here, even better than what you could have imagined, so be grateful for once!' She held her head like it was going to explode.

I worked myself stupid to cover up what I was feeling. Two weeks before we were to wed, I finally decided to face up to what I was feeling. I had a huge weight upon me. I was exhausted as I'd been unable to sleep and I sat in our study at sunrise one day and felt this grief rush over me, an enormous sense of paranoia and fear. I had everything at my feet and all I had to do was trust in the process, be that young woman who expected everything and got everything she asked for – a princess, a queen – but all I felt like was a complete and utter phony.

I was lost over which path to take in my life. I was panicked because I'd started to have second thoughts about marrying

Charlie. My mind's voice was telling me I was making a huge mistake and I was repeating to myself, *Don't do it, don't go ahead with this. Don't do this to him and you, you will be so unhappy. Don't do it*. It was so loud. Then I would answer myself. *But you can't. You bought a house. You have a business together. Oh my God, you have two dogs. Who will get the dogs? We can't split them up; they'll be so upset*. It replayed over and over.

That box I had in my brain that I'd shoved so many past experiences into? Well, it was starting to make rumbling noises and I could hear distant warning bells.

Finally, after work one night, I decided to face my internal ugliness, sit down and approach it like an adult – something I had not done before, ever. I asked Charlie to sit down with me. I calmly spoke about my fears, expressing what I felt were my serious concerns. He needed to know the truth. I poured my heart and soul out, and I couldn't have been clearer, more levelheaded. It didn't go as planned.

He begged me not to back out of the wedding. He pleaded, saying his family would never forgive him. Then he started crying, which made it worse.

I couldn't believe it. I needed him to listen to me, but it wasn't to be. I had so many things that were going around in my mind but it was to no avail. So I decided to avoid them. Lowering my head into my hands I gave up. I walked into the kitchen, picked a bottle of red from the selection we had in a cheap wooden wine holder and a glass and went out into the backyard with the dogs.

'Where are you going? Are you leaving me now?' His soft-pitched voice ground on my nerves. It wasn't even the voice of a man, more a boy. 'Don't drink like that, Jack. Your doctor warned you.'

'Charles, please leave me alone. I kindly listened to you now kindly reciprocate and listen to me. Piss off.'

I didn't understand that there could be an exchange of dialogue, that something so important could be discussed. I didn't mean that he was wrong or that I was at fault – logically both sides should have been considered, but they weren't. It wasn't two adults dealing with life; it was two kids. One trying to run away out of projected fear and another fearful of what his family thought.

I could distinctly feel something was very off. What was happening in my gut, a feeling in the pit of my stomach, was very similar to how I felt on the grounds of the Kew Asylum. I could strongly feel my instinct but I chose to ignore it because I was going to make him unhappy. I didn't want to upset him or our families. Again, I snuffed it out.

I'm definitely a believer in signs, markers to look out for to guide you through life. But I completely ignored them when I was about to walk down the aisle. I instead took the route to please others on the Disneyland express, where girl meets boy, boy proposes, they get married in some over-the-top romantic ritual where they offer their lives to one another under the premise that no one else could fulfil their desires and then melt comfortably into the suburban dream.

The signs were there when I look back now with a sober perspective.

Three days before the wedding, I was called by one of my future sister-in-laws. She proceeded to tell me that her and her younger sister had tried on their bridesmaid dresses for their mother and she, in her infinite, perfect wisdom, had decided they didn't look right so proceeded to unpick the hems then cut them with scissors. She told me they were seeing a better seamstress that afternoon and everything would be fine. I bit my tongue and thanked her for letting me know.

When we were getting our photos taken as a bridal party, Bob, one of Charlie's groomsmen launched into a hilarious story that they were all in a car accident before they got to the wedding.

'It's OK, Jack. The guys who ran into us gave us a lift, so it's not like we were late. So funny,' he said.

My jaw hit the ground, as I didn't see the irony. Little did they know, I felt like the whole event was a complete car crash. I'm sure the photographer got a shot of it. They say that photographers are very blessed with the sense of seeing which couples would last in matrimony. I often wondered if he could see trouble ahead.

Just before Dad walked me down the aisle we stood, arms linked, at the entrance to the beautiful native garden before us. I turned to him, told him I loved him and had decided to keep my maiden name. Looking back, it was a declaration of my love to him. All I wanted was for him to show me the scarcest offering that he cared. It didn't happen. His response was given through gritted teeth and a beaming smile, as he knew people were staring at us.

'I don't give a shit. You're not my problem anymore.'

He'd sold his business to Charlie and I and got what he'd wanted, end of story. And again, I was left standing next to a narcissistic individual whose attention I craved, hurt and embarrassed by his behaviour. Our relationship was predictable; I was needy and he was an arsehole.

And to finish it off …

The night of our wedding, after wearing a beautiful, tailored gown and a mask of love and contentment for seven hours in a stunning setting, Charlie and I returned to our bridal suite. The room was covered in one hundred dollar bills and cheques that totalled over 10,000 dollars. It was the tradition of Charlie's family background. The thought process was that a big money gift to the wedded couple proved your worth as a friend to the parents. I lay in the darkness of our marital bed with my new husband, consummating our union. I felt so alone and warm tears rolled down my cheeks. I dared not make a noise either as it would bring attention that I didn't want. All I could think of was what a mistake I had just made, even though I had received everything I had originally wished for. It was another event to put in the box. Instead of feeling giddy with excitement over our planned future together, all I could think was, *What the hell have I just done?*

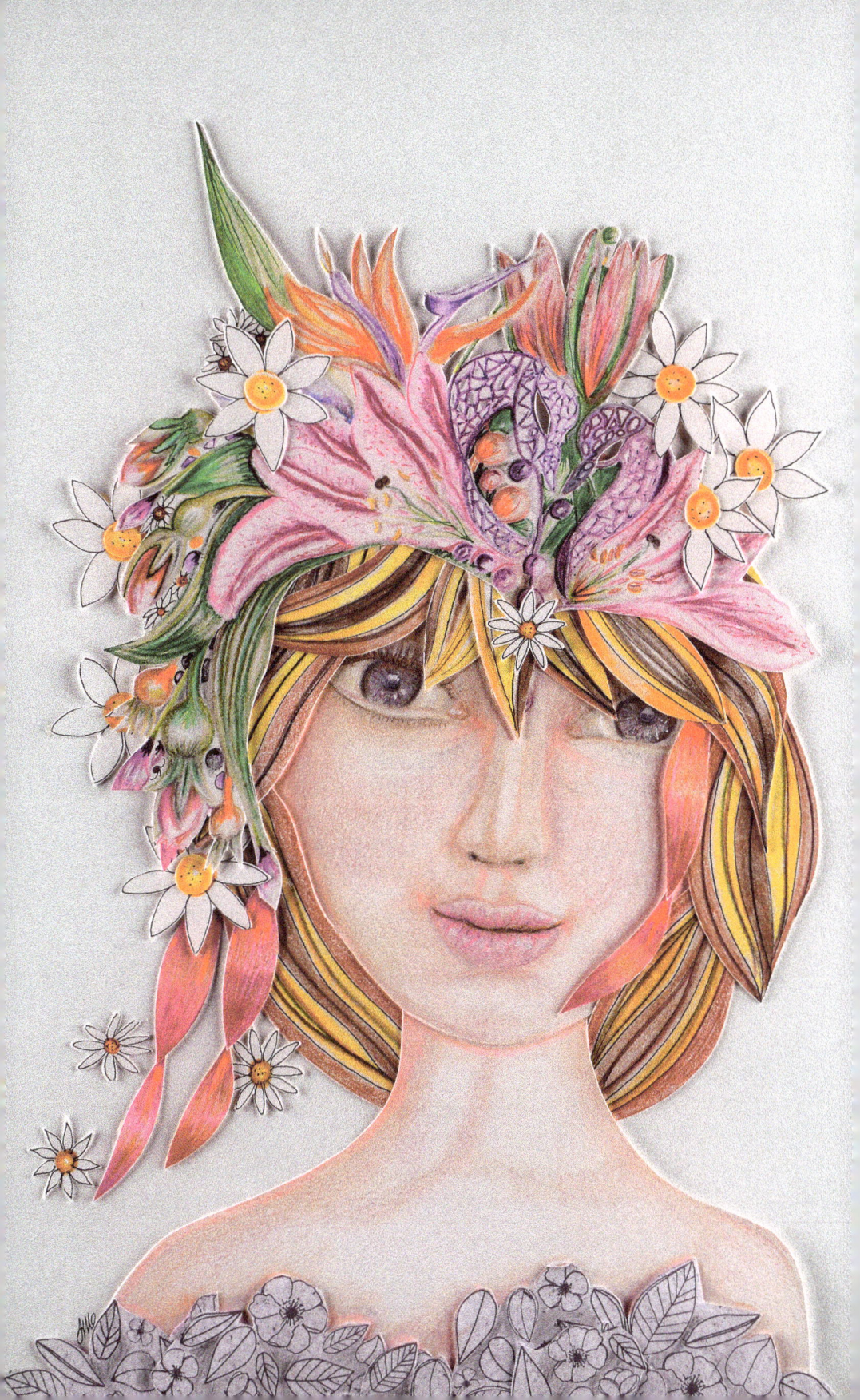

1997

After cutting our honeymoon short from ten nights to four due to being uncomfortable in my new husband's company, I returned to my day job as a manager. On the first Thursday night trade since I had come back, I sent two of my staff members off to get their dinner at the same time, as it had been a quiet day.

I was the only remaining person within the store and what occurred next got the ball rolling to a point where my mind couldn't cope any further. Trust me when I say it was painful but necessary.

As I stood inside the shop and behind the oval-shaped counter reading some notes from morning meetings with supervisors, a group of eight to ten youths in their early teens, boys and girls, merged on the shop all at once. One of the boys jumped the counter and brandished a knife at my face, while his mates ripped a laptop out of the back wall. I wanted to tell him to put the knife down but I closed my eyes, frozen with fear.

Back in 1996 sleek looking laptops were new in Australia and were highly expensive. These kids did a snatch and grab, but talk about a butterfly effect. It was a catalyst for another adjustment in my life.

For one slight moment in time, they were in the shop and the next they weren't. It wasn't unlike being attacked in the city. Within an instant my life changed. I was stunned as to what I had just been a part of. On autopilot, I ran to the roller door, pulled it down, locked it, and then I called security. In the meantime, my staff had returned from their break and I had to recount the story to them, but I did it in an extremely controlled way. I couldn't let anyone know how I was feeling inside. In my mind there was that little voice yelling out that I wasn't allowed to embarrass myself. Security finally turned up and told me they'd found the gang on their security footage but lost them in the huge shopping centre we worked in.

I called my area supervisor and state manager, but they refused to get the police involved. It was all way too much for me to deal with but I kept my perfect mask on so to those outside I looked cool and calm. I responded to all the questioning, and then around 10 pm, after taking a call from Charlie asking where I was, my state manager escorted me to my car. He placed his large hands on my shoulders and, looking directly into my eyes, told me not to worry about it.

'It happens all the time, Jack. Don't worry about it. Go home and sleep it off. Night.'

That was the company's way of counselling; it was delivered in seconds.

I drove the fifteen minutes it took to get home, stepped out of my car, walked inside and collapsed on the lounge room floor. My legs just gave way. Charlie was waiting up for me, and watched in horror as I hit the ground. I recall him getting on the ground to comfort me but I didn't want to be touched; I just wanted to be left alone. Eventually he assisted me in getting to bed, but I didn't leave it for three days. I didn't eat or drink – nothing. I felt paralysed with fear and I fell in and out of a deep, protective sleep. There were several times though when I did open my eyes and there was an elderly lady sitting at the end of my bed, but I wasn't scared. She just watched me from Charlie's side of the bed.

'Who is she? Did you call someone to look after me? I don't need her,' I asked Charlie. I was infuriated he'd told someone. I was embarrassed and just want to be invisible.

'No, princess, I'd never do that. There's no one here. Just get better, you'll be ok.' He was soothing me by rubbing the doona to get me back to sleep. It was the only time I felt protected. Sleep and alcohol or alcohol and then sleep – my two best friends.

Charlie had spoken with my staff to find out in length what I'd been witness to but professional counselling was never offered to me, let alone medical assistance in getting something to calm my nerves. I was a child to a generation of parents where you just got on with things. I was told that if I did return I would be posted to another of the company's shops, much further away from where I lived. They weren't making it easier for me, but harder. The company's internal philosophy was to get me to be quiet due to the impact the robbery had on me. To them I was a WorkCover liability waiting to happen.

Charlie told work I would be returning but he couldn't tell them when as I couldn't face leaving the house. I just couldn't comprehend why those kids had done what they had. Again, I was left asking why. What had I done wrong? Over and over. But no one's answers softened the anxiety I was feeling.

It was then decided I had to leave my marriage.

I had to get away from home. Home wasn't safe; I had to run away. I didn't trust anyone, so I packed my car with some basics while Charlie was at work and drove to my cousin's house, but I couldn't outrun the anxiety travelling through me. I was petrified. What I didn't realise was that it was not just the shop hold-up that was upsetting me; it was the whole package of my life that was dark and black. I felt that I had failed in everything. I felt no one wanted to listen to me and, as I had been abused again and again, my mind couldn't cope. Fear and anger circulated in my mind constantly.

At my cousin's home, an hour from where Charlie and I lived, I slept on his couch and when awake I drank. I was lucky to have Teddy looking over me. I trusted him, as he'd never expected anything from me. After tracking me down, Dad got on the phone and told me in no uncertain terms I was a complete disgrace to the family again and if I did not get home to my husband immediately, he would cut me off from speaking to Mum and my sisters.

'You have a husband to look after and business to run with him. Get the fuck home now.'

I couldn't handle the thought of not seeing them, so I dried out and reluctantly returned to Charlie. Once home I tried to explain to him what I thought was going on but again it fell on deaf ears. He just gently told me I had had a nervous breakdown, then said, 'But, princess, I want you to look on the bright side, maybe see it as a breakthrough not a breakdown!' There was soft music playing in the background, so he put his arms around me and we rocked gently. He tenderly sang and I cried into his chest, ready to concede. Breakthrough about what? Could nobody else see it?

The insidious chatter in my head was so loud and the negative self-talk was obtrusively repetitive. I'd be constantly waking up in the middle of the night, pacing the house, worried about what other people thought about me and in fear that I was going to be attacked again. It was paranoia beyond belief and it was shocking. My skin bled from scratching my scalp – if I bled there no one could see how insane I felt. Blackness was rising up in my throat – I couldn't speak. I'd race to the toilet and throw up, then rest my forehead on the edge of the cold bowl, quietly crying. I couldn't let Charlie hear when he was asleep, as he'd try and pacify me again and I didn't need soothing. I needed to scream, I needed out, I needed help. I desperately wanted direction as to what to do next but there was nothing but emptiness. I'd been raised to listen for my next instruction but none came. I wanted someone to be out there waiting for me, to tell me what to do.

It was not to be the last time I left Charlie either. I packed my car and left our home three times before he decided to sell our business and move us interstate. He hoped that I would feel better with a change of surrounds and more sun. I was pretty sure it wasn't a lack of vitamin D that was causing my grief. I asked him time and again for a divorce but he just ignored me and I felt that I had to have his approval to do it, just as I had always needed my parents' approval to do anything in life. I suppose I was going to have to learn the hard way, and I did.

1998

Acclaimed American psychiatrist Dr Gordon Livingston wrote a chapter in his book *Too Soon Old, Too Late Smart* titled 'We are all prone to the myth of the perfect stranger'.

When I read it, I found that it struck a chord in describing how I felt whilst I was married to Charlie. It reads:

'No element of dissatisfaction with our lives is more common than the belief that we have in our youth made the wrong choice of partner. The fantasies generated therefore often take the form of a conversation that there exists somewhere the person who will save us with his or her love. Much of the infidelity that is the hallmark of unhappy marriages rests on this illusion.'

I was never unfaithful to Charlie but I seriously considered it, unconsciously thinking it would be the easy way out. Thankfully some sanity must have remained, as I just couldn't do it to him.

But the thought of being saved never left my mind. The feeling never left that there was that perfect someone out there who would fix everything for me, someone who was stronger and wiser, someone who I could hand my grief to and they would make it disappear. I was becoming very aggravated and so Charlie tried everything he could to fix what he really could not fix, as it wasn't his pain.

I was so uninspired to do anything either way. It was like catching a train to somewhere but I never knew where we'd end up, I didn't care. I was merely a passenger and had completely disconnected with myself.

Our dogs were flown up to Queensland to meet us and we started our road trip to a brighter future, a new beginning, a happy ending, and if you believe that then you're insane. I knew in my heart that moving was not the answer, but never spoke a word. We were merely extending the inevitable. I just smiled and waved Mum goodbye one April morning. Again, I allowed someone to make a major decision in my life and I said nothing.

It didn't take long for both of us to find work once we arrived. I landed a managerial role with the Hyatt hotel group. Work was not keeping me happy so I decided to do something that did. I shopped. I decided that we needed a new house, so it was built, surrounded by a tropical garden, and so it was landscaped. I decorated the house with new furniture that looked so gorgeous it ended up being photographed for an ad in *Home Beautiful*.

I was in a hollow existence. Every night I drank to excess and when I was conscious I'd plan how I was going to spend money. My paranoia never left – it was mine and I naively owned it. Being in my head was delusional so to just keep moving forward drinking and spending was my answer.

When I returned to Melbourne for a surprise visit for Mum on her seventieth birthday, I found out to my absolute surprise that I was pregnant. It was something else to keep my brain occupied, even though Charlie and I never wanted children to begin with. We wanted to remain the 1990s acronym of DINKs: Double Income No Kids.

As soon as I returned to Queensland, though, I was so happy to tell him our exciting news. He was dumbfounded and I was to miscarry six weeks into the pregnancy. After that letdown something else was conjuring up inside my mind: I started to consider taking my own life. It came to a point where I was discussing with Charlie who I thought he should date or marry if I was not to be around any longer. He ignored my banter as just that, nothing serious.

For some reason that I understand now but didn't then, my relationship with Charlie after the miscarriage became more like a brother/sister one to me than a husband-and-wife union. I couldn't even stomach the thought of sex anymore. At his request we visited a psychologist who specialised in sexual relationships. For our first piece of homework I was asked to just hold Charlie in the hope it would rekindle something that was once there ... I couldn't even allow him to look at me with that thought in mind, let alone touch him.

I'd even placed the number of the local brothel on speed dial for him if he wanted sex. I told him that if he felt like having it,

I wouldn't stand in his way of visiting the local establishment. He never took up the offer though. He told me he loved only me and due to being stressed sex was the last thing on his mind. Thank goodness we had something in common.

During work one afternoon I went to the human resources division and asked a couple of the other managers to write me references. I told them I needed the letters as I was renting a place of my own as Charlie and I were splitting up. I had a few rostered days off so I decided to take the letters and activate another one of my hair-brain ideas. I went down to one of the local real estate agents with my credit card and my references. I signed a six-month contract for a townhouse. Erratically driving home, I packed my car with some basics and left Charlie a note telling him where I was. I was running away again, with a palpable and overwhelming feeling I had to leave.

Once there, in an extreme state of excitement, I furnished the apartment over the next few days with little sleep. I was living on adrenalin, another manic episode, but I only lasted a week until I became so overcome with depression. I had to call Charlie, as I knew I was in trouble. Immediately after calling him, I laid down on the bare carpet and fell into a deep sleep. I was woken by my mobile phone ringing. It was Charlie, and he was outside the apartment. I was so disorientated I had a panic attack and burst into tears – I couldn't work out where I was. The apartment manager let Charlie into the apartment. He drove me to our local doctor where she recommended that, as we had private health insurance, he should drive me as soon as possible to Belmont Private Hospital in Brisbane.

Belmont is the largest mental health hospital in Queensland, situated ten kilometres outside of Brisbane and where I was to reside for the following six weeks. Soon after my arrival I was booked in to undergo the first of twelve treatments of ECT or electroconvulsive therapy. My appointed psychiatrist had diagnosed me for the first time with manic depressive disorder and had started me on course of lithium.

I'm going to save you Googling it.

Electroconvulsive therapy is a psychiatric treatment where seizures are electrically induced in patients to provide relief from mental disorders. Basically the only thing they didn't do was put me in a straitjacket.

I didn't understand what I was about to put myself through, to put my mind through, my body. It was truly debilitating as it took my short-term memory away, which later angered me greatly as I have always had a very clear memory. After ECT it took me years to recall events that were previously crystal clear. I was so frustrated that I couldn't even recall certain family member's names for up to three months after.

Anne called me from Melbourne truly concerned and asked how I was feeling before my first treatment. She wanted to know if I understood the seriousness of it all. I told her in a very disconnected state that I was tired of it all. I didn't care anymore. It wasn't so much the statement of a victim; I was just ready to concede to everything. I was going to go along with whatever the doctor wanted, whatever Charlie wanted.

Mum flew up from Melbourne and stayed in the local motel across the road two weeks before I was to leave hospital. She sat by my bedside every day. She kept me company when I wasn't in CBT or the therapy group that included all types of people, from anorexics, to mums with post-natal depression and people with schizophrenia – the whole team was there.

I could at least say that I felt safe where I was. I felt protected from the outside world, as things had started to become unpredictable for me. I couldn't trust myself or how I'd react to everyday happenings. The irony was that some of the group members insisted they were worse mentally than any of the others and loved letting everyone know. Then there were others who didn't give a shit either way. It was quite literally a complete mad house.

I smoked and drank coffee all day to keep me awake from all the sedatives and watched life go by. I knew there was something seriously wrong but I kept quiet and kept my head down, hoping not to bring attention to myself. I tried my hardest to keep the perfect mask on, not allowing anyone really inside to see what had happened in the past.

When my visit was coming to an end and I was not seen as a suicide risk anymore, I was allowed out from the hospital some mornings with Mum. We went to the local shopping centre to see how I'd cope going back into the community. We'd go to the cinema and watch a movie. I loved just sitting in a darkened room and I'm sure we caught some great movies, but due to the ECT I completely forgot them as soon as I had my next treatment. I may have seen the same movie four times – I have no idea. It was irony at its best.

When I finally returned back up state it was Christmas. I don't recall much of Christmas Day and even after daily medication, six weeks of ECT, CBT and talking daily to my appointed psychiatrist I still never spoke a word about what Dad did when I was a kid, being attacked in the city or even the most recent event of the robbery. It didn't register as important because everyone else seemed to just blow it off and get on with their lives. What was the use? I couldn't see what was right in front of my eyes, or I should say behind my eyes. Inside my brain, I had become a casualty in my own mind. I still felt that if I could just leave my marriage I would feel better. I mean, it couldn't hurt to try again and ask for a reprieve. Thank God I was finally granted my wish.

After leaving Charlie four times I was given the wonderful opportunity to leave him for the fifth and final time when his mother and sisters came up to visit us after my mum had left. I wanted to be left alone so basically locked myself in our bedroom, slept or read for two weeks through the disgusting, tropical muggy heat that Queensland had to offer.

Once his family finally left Charlie angrily spoke those golden words I'd been longing to hear since the night we wed.

'Jackie, you were so rude to my family. That's it. I want a divorce.'

Really? That was all I had to do? Sit in our bedroom for two weeks and be glaringly unsociable? Hell, if I'd known that I would have tried it much sooner.

I responded immediately. 'OK.'

He picked up speed so I let him rant and scream at the top of his voice, which was very unusual for him to do. Since we'd been together, Charlie had only gotten angry once prior to this outburst. On the Richter scale this tantrum came in at maybe eight out of ten but I was prepared to accept it immediately so I fell on my sword. I pretended I was listening to him, nodding my head, agreeing that I'd completely ruined his life, our marriage and even that of our dogs.

Once he paused for a breath, I asked to use the phone. 'Hold that thought, I've just got to make a call.'

He started at me, confused.

Dialling Mum interstate, I told her I was coming home on the next flight available. Charlie then continued his rant, threatening that I wouldn't get a single penny from him. I silenced him quickly as I agreed. 'I don't want anything from you ... all I need to do is go home, to be left alone. That's all I'm asking for.'

My only request was that I could take what furniture I brought into the marriage even though when I was well I'd been paying the mortgage to the house and business.

In the end he got the house, the dogs – everything except my car and I can't even remember why I asked for that. Materialistically I gave away everything because it meant nothing to me. I felt so empty and nothing tangible had meaning to me anymore.

I returned to Melbourne and unconsciously allowed my parents to take over again, even organising legal advice for me. My parents' lawyer, Erica, was ready to rip Charlie apart, limb from limb. I was mentally and physically exhausted and couldn't be bothered putting him or myself through the legal system after seven years of what I felt like was water torture. Charlie had put up with so much through my illness and if I could have done anything right at least I was going to leave him as swiftly as possible without any legal implications so he could get on with his life. He was a good person but I couldn't deal with living with a 'good husband'. I also couldn't stand the thought of making an enemy of him. If I'd fought it legally I would have easily walked away with well over 100,000 dollars in the bank but I just didn't have the energy nor could I do it to him. Seven years to the day that we wed, I countersigned our divorce papers. A perfect execution of the seven-year itch.

Charlie's father wrote me a letter expressing his thoughts on our split union. He was to remove my name from the title of the house therefore releasing me of any responsibility to repay the mortgage.

> ... I have always and still think very highly of you and sincerely hope you recover with the help and support from your loving parents. Please feel free to call us any time at home or the office. You will always be welcome in my home. If I can be of any assistance in any way do not hesitate to contact me. We would like to have you over for dinner when you feel well enough to attend.
>
> For now, receive our best wishes.
>
> Love, Bernard.

Charlie's father was one of Melbourne's most revered solicitors and apart from being not of sound mind, well, deep down I knew I didn't have a chance for calm separation had he become involved. It could have gotten very ugly.

Once back in Melbourne and under my parents' roof, I realised that I was seeing the same pattern: parents drinking, fighting and running my life. I didn't know how to outrun it, I didn't know a better way, I couldn't see how it could change, I didn't know I had a choice. I was resigned to the fact that it was my lot in life.

I had to return to Queensland one last time to get a few basic furniture pieces onto a removal truck but the night before I got on the plane everything erupted in my mind again.

Mum hadn't done anything to deserve being in the direct line of psychotic rage but I snapped, unable to explain why. One minute we were talking about nothing in particular and then I had a rush of panic run through me. I started trying to pick a fight with her, which I never did. I never spoke back to my parents, but I just exploded. It was pure panic.

'You fucking bitch. I'm going to kill you!' I was enraged.

I picked up the closest thing I could find, a solid amber glass ashtray, and threw it at her head. My action was so quick. Thank

God I missed her head but it was only by centimetres. The glass shattered into hundreds of pieces as it hit the brick wall she was standing in front of, thick glass shards showering her.

It was pure hysteria. An enormous amount of grief was flooding me. Anne had just arrived to have dinner with us and before I knew it she was pulling me into her car and driving me away from the house to protect me from Dad. He was left to comfort Mum from my shocking actions. Once at Anne's I fell into another deep sleep, waking early the following morning to catch a taxi to Tullamarine to fly back to Queensland.

I received a call from my father a few days later telling me that I was never to return to their house.

'We're absolutely horrified by your shocking behaviour. It's out of control and you will never be allowed back here ever again, Jack. *Ever*. You are on your own.'

The line went dead.

I didn't blame him, but I couldn't explain my actions. To do so would mean I'd have had to understand what had happened to me over years and I didn't even know what I'd been through was damaging. I was at a complete loss.

Now, I didn't have anywhere to live in Melbourne, so I stayed in one of the spare bedrooms at Charlie's for three weeks. My main source of nourishment was from mainly alcohol and nicotine. I knew I had to face my family and it horrified me what I'd left behind when I attacked Mum. I had to get back though, so getting an upgrade to business class on my Qantas flight back to Melbourne was a sign in my mind for me to live it up. I'd officially become homeless and I'd be living in my car so it was booze all the way until touchdown.

Anne picked me up from the gate and I was wired. It was an alcoholic state where I had a sense I was high but truly felt my guise was solid. It wasn't.

2001

I'll let my eldest sister Anne explain:

'I'd been living with my boyfriend Conner, who I am now married to, for only a month, when we went to the airport to pick Jackie up after her final trip to Queensland. I thought I was emotionally prepared. After all, she'd had the recommended treatment of ECT, and been away to get herself together. I thought surely she was pretty much her old self and things would improve from now on. How wrong was I.

'When I saw her walking quickly towards me along the gateway, it was clear something was very askew. Her eyes were overly bright, cheeks flushed, and she was very thin. Her gorgeous big smile was there, but an odd, somewhat distorted version, the sort of smile you get when the muscles and skin stretch in the usual and expected manner but your inner emotions are anything but happy.

'Her arms were flapping around like a distressed bird and she was talking just about nonstop. As it turns out, on top of the multiple prescribed medications, she had drunk to calm her nerves on the plane. Her responses and behaviour were garish, arms flailing, voice loud, harsh like jagged glass, unexpected. She was talking and talking and talking, laughing and talking again.

'As we approached the baggage carousel, a short, very well-known millionaire and former doctor Geoffrey Edelstein hurried forward to grab his bag. "Doctor E," cried Jack, as though he was her long-lost friend.

'She grabbed his hand and shook it so hard I thought he would lift off the ground. She told him how wonderful it was to finally meet him. The poor, startled medic handled the assault on his personal space with surprising aplomb for a man of his stature and reputation, and then dashed off the moment she released him. It was comical and disturbing all at once. Jack kept talking and talking, who knows what about, so much so that we became distracted and forgot one of her bags. We had to go back the next day.

'Due to not being able to go back to our parents, she stayed with us for a week or so. After the alcohol and nerves wore off, she plunged. I was left looking at my sister, the energy so negative that I could almost see the blackness emanating from her small frame. Endless negative energy. It was truly awful.

'If I have depression it's mild and usually in response to external events. I have gained relief from CBT, meditation and the like. But Jackie's struggle with her mind is a whole other story.

'Picture this: you walk into a room where your beloved sister is sitting. This is the baby sister you held, completely adored from the moment she was bought home, played with, laughed with. A sister with who your memories are filled with happy experiences.

'Now she becomes so distressed that she cries most of the time, and not just quiet crying, but deep shuddering cries filled with despair that go on and on. She sleeps much of the day as a relief from feeling. She is constantly cold despite the sunny weather, cannot eat, grows thinner each day and when she's lying on the couch, she appears to be simply a bundle of clothes from which that deathly black energy continues to push outwards. Looking at her I always had an image of this energy being so negative that it had the power to reveal a deep, icy, bottomless cavern, where no light could penetrate.

'We never knew this would be only one of many extreme tortuous cycles that Jack would have to go through, different life experiences that she wasn't able to cope with. The years have seen her go up and down many times and through many different life experiences. In hindsight, it's clear that her mental troubles started long before that first crisis period.'

And then there's Jane's version:

'It wasn't until Jackie's first marriage started falling apart that we all really saw the first signs of serious depressive illness. When she stayed with my family when she couldn't return to our parents, she told me one day that she'd sit on the couch and look at the clock – four hours would go by and she wouldn't remember any of it. She lost days with no memory of them occurring.

'Our family as a whole, like a lot of people at the time, didn't know how to deal with depression and we tried to support her the best we could, whilst getting on with our own busy lives. She struggled for years. Multiple doctors, multiple medications, stints in hospital, it was a rollercoaster and not just for her but the rest of us. It was so draining and, after staying with Anne, she spent a few nights in her car. Then I was able to get her into our home for a few weeks, even though it took a lot of convincing. She was just lost.

'It was exhausting and I do remember sometimes removing myself from the circus in her mind which she lived in to keep myself sane. My husband could see me struggling when she stayed and he was my biggest support. We were raising our sons and having Jack with our family was as though I had an extra child to look after. She was an adult and it was more difficult to live with her than the three teenagers that we had. She didn't have any "true south"; she was an empty rudderless ship.

'As difficult as it has been, though, I have never stopped loving her. But her illness was shocking and I didn't know how to deal with it. I was there but I didn't know how to help her – none of us did. That's my biggest regret. I didn't know how to help her.'

For over four months I'd been placed on a cocktail of medication including lithium and it wasn't doing anything remotely positive for me. Looking back, it was as though I had so much baggage from my past history to deal with. Until I faced up to it, it morphed into truly ugly behaviour that I could no longer live with, let alone any of my family.

Now if you've gotten to this point in the book and are screaming blue murder and wanting to bang your head against a wall because you can see the pattern well and truly – that's a bit how my friends and family felt. But I couldn't see it. I was welded to the manic ups and detrimental downs as a natural part of my existence. It was a victim state of affairs but I wasn't of sound mind to rectify the situation.

It was ten years later when I was in a domestic violence survivor group that a light bulb went off. One of the reasons I felt so uncomfortable and unwilling to give my first marriage a chance was because after the abuse I had lived with I couldn't recognise a healthy relationship with anyone, male or female, if it were to fall on me. In his nature Charlie was giving and kind and I found it repulsive to a point where I couldn't live with him, no matter how hard he tried to make it better. It sickened me to be in his company.

In regards to going through the ECT, I have feelings of regret and sadness that well up inside me when I realise what I put myself through. At the time I was so lost and desperate. Still to this day if I get overly stressed once asleep, I'll be woken with a feeling of an electric current running through my body, as though I'm feeling a shock. Medical professionals say that due to a general anaesthetic being administered prior to the commencement of treatment you won't be able to recall the actual event, but someone forgot to tell my subconscious that.

2001 – September

After a few weeks of living with and ultimately wearing my stay out with Jane via exhaustion (hers not mine), I was allowed to return to Mum and Dad's. But only under one rule: I had to agree I would see another psychiatrist. They even insisted on driving me to prove to themselves I was actually attending.

I agreed and was placed on another medication. Bipolar was ruled out even though my behaviour was truly erratic. Lithium wasn't working on me. There was obviously a golden rule within the Psychiatric Golden Rule Textbook that states, 'If your patient does not respond to lithium chloride then they will not have bipolar'.

Towards the middle of September 2001, something very special happened.

I had a conversation with a woman on the phone who had called my workplace looking to purchase a product that my brother-in-law Andrew stocked in his business. Thinking nothing of it, she said that she would drive over and pick it up. A few hours later that woman came into my workplace and it turned out to be none other than my long-lost best friend Clair. She was pregnant and was holding the hand of a small child who was her first-born son.

I couldn't believe it. I had heard that Clair had gone overseas to Europe five years previously but we had lost contact. She kindly asked me up for a cup of tea at her home that afternoon and I had the pleasure of meeting her husband, William. We clicked back into place straight away and I was so grateful for many reasons. One that really stood out was I knew Clair's family were members of a local church that I had attended a few times with her as a teenager and I was interested if they still attended. They did.

Feeling as lost as I was, I felt it was time to connect with something bigger than myself, something that maybe could bring me the peace I yearned for. That's what I thought religion could do for me. To me it seemed Clair had always been on the right track. I admired her parents greatly as they were so supportive of their daughter, and family was a big focus of the church. I started attending on Sundays with Clair and at the start it gave me a strong sense of positive guidance. I thought for a short time too that my new medication had started to make me feel better. I found that I was feeling more able to start socialising a bit more.

One day I took up an offer from a guy called Scott who used to come into work. He asked me if I wanted to go out for a drink one night with some friends of his. He seemed a nice enough guy so I thought why not. Looking back I wish I had asked 'Why?' and then decided not.

Once out, I found out that I liked his cheeky personality and I matched it, line for line. He was a good-looking bloke, a four-wheel driving tradie. On the weekends if he wasn't riding around on his Ducati motorbike, he would be up bush with mates, shooting wild pigs. OK, so we had absolutely nothing in common, but being a professional chameleon of personalities, I knew I would fit in perfectly, eventually, somehow. I would find a way. I came from a safe marriage with a 'good boy'. Even though I was attending church there was a much greater pull in that I was ready to have some real fun. When Scott arrived on the scene, I got shown the ultimate 'bad boy' and decided to grab it with both hands, and I hung on very tightly. I proceeded to stray from the safety of friends, family and medication. It was as if I was living a double life: good girl on a Sunday and during the day at work, but at night I was ready to party hard, and we did.

Adrenaline is an amazing tool when your mind and body are flooded with it. But then the flip side became apparent after too many weeks of exhausting late nights. That's when I'd be back in a bad headspace again, pushing towards major depression. That commanded me to mask everything I was feeling when in public. This cycle just added to what I felt was the excitement of it all. Stupidly, I decided to let Scott know about my medication for depression.

He'd been witness to how exciting, provocative, crazy and fun I could be and took it as my 'normal', which wasn't the truth. I couldn't keep that behaviour up on a 24-hour cycle so I put on that 'mask' each time we met. I played the role of a person he wanted me to be, sprinkled with a hint of another of my favourites – the Nice Girl. I was a bit of everything I thought he'd like a woman to be.

I had a constant feeling that I had to be an open book to everyone. I believed that if I was fun, honest and nice then surely everyone else would be nice to me, right? I pivoted on the assumptions of others as though daily changing of perceptions was the norm. Whatever was needed, I was the answer. Whatever was then said, I made it my new mantra. I handed over everything that makes a person whole. I completely lost my way but I was convinced that someone else who was a complete stranger had all the answers. My life became a mush of counterfactual behaviour but I pushed through with such drive, hedging my bets that I'd fall on my feet and everything would come back around in perfect sequence to benefit me.

In this frame of mind, it didn't take too much effort for Scott to convince me that he'd be there for me. He wanted me to go off my meds, much to my physiatrist's horror. He literally begged me not to make such a rash decision based on a stranger's opinion that wasn't based on supporting me. It resulted in me telling the good doctor that I didn't need him anymore, along with the medication. I was ready to take on the world. That, my dear reader, is not called being confident, but merely delusional.

For the first time in my life, I rode on the back of a motorbike in a summer dress, bare feet, without a helmet, at high speed on the back roads of country towns. I was taught how to shoot a rifle – thank goodness only at clay pigeons. Adding to this blossoming warped relationship was being taken to a gun club and taught how to use handgun, very romantic indeed. I would have fitted into Trump World beautifully had it been nineteen years earlier. The wonderful combination of using firearms while being mentally unstable – it was a beautiful thing until I hit a wall.

I hadn't up to that point been rational and realised who I was dating. Well, it did cross my mind but it never dawned on me what he was actually capable of. I always gave him the benefit of the doubt. Every time.

One Sunday afternoon, after a 4WD session with about five of Scott's friends in country Victoria, we'd woven our way through paddocks to arrive at an abandoned house. I sat under a large gumtree, trying to keep cool, as the day's temperature was in the high thirties. All of a sudden, I felt a sharp pain and heard a hard clunk: Scott had deliberately knocked the back of my skull with the barrel of his shotgun, which I'd just witnessed him load. He stood in front of me, pointing the shotgun directly at my face. Within a spilt second, he lowered the rifle. My head dropped in fear. He then raised it again, aiming at the tree canopy.

The horror of having my head blown off was replaced by the sound of a deafening shotgun blast. I was cowering on the ground, screaming, with a mangled magpie and fragments of a nest landing on me. Scott had killed a mother magpie that had been sitting on her young above my head. It was official. I was dating a psychopath.

I couldn't have told you then that he did it for a laugh from his mates because I was petrified. Did he want to shoot me? No, I don't believe he did, but his actions and behaviour were appalling and my reaction was immediate. I went into autopilot. I froze. Instead of showing him I was horrified and angry I took the other route. I made excuses for his behaviour. Was he showing off in front of his mates? Maybe he'd had too much to drink, because guns and alcohol normally always mix. I was stuck on a property with an irrational man who had a loaded gun so if I was ever going to portray anything other than scared now was the time.

Those undeniable red flags had been showing themselves for weeks, but I'd ignored them. He was using cocaine, and I started noticing his mate's poor behaviour towards their partners and wives. He also began putting me down in front of his friends for a laugh at my expense. Even small things like cancelling dates or not turning up after we had made a time to meet. Today it would be called 'ghosting'. Back then it was called 'where the fuck is he?'

I was completely confused and looked forward to a slight morsel of attention. My mind looked for what I had done to deserve this behaviour rather than thinking his behaviour was wrong and not that of someone I wanted to be with.

After the shooting, when we were all finally back on the road, the feeling of absolute shame and humiliation engulfed me, but I stayed straight-faced and silent. Once back at Scott's property, everyone was starting to drink. I quietly made my exit so no one could notice me. My ears were still ringing from the blast and I had adrenalin running through me but I also wanted to shut down. I tried to steady my breathing and told myself to get home. My head ached and was throbbing from the blow I'd received from the gun. A thought popped into my mind that if I told Mum she'd just as likely say, 'It was just a gun, don't worry about it, just let it go. Stop taking everything so personally'. It was then I surrendered to the fact I'd never mention the incident to anyone. Not to my family or my girlfriends, let alone the police. Scott had mates in the force and so to me it wasn't worth it; I wasn't worth it. I buried it again.

I was completely humiliated to such an extent that I threw up in the garden when I got home. Thank God my parents weren't home. My head throbbed terribly; my throat was acidic from vomiting. I made my way into the shower and sat on the floor and sobbed. Shame engulfed me.

Finally, I got out. Wrapping a towel around me but not even drying myself, I went into the lounge room and found a bottle of Scotch my parents had on hand for guests. I opened it and started drinking straight from the bottle. After finally feeling its effect, I headed to bed and passed out.

The saddest thing of all was that once I awoke the next morning with an aching head, I wanted to go back to Scott's house and apologise. Apologise for triggering his reaction with something I may have done, anything – I had to be at fault. My ego ached from being discarded – I'd fucked up again. I was mortified at the position I put myself in, then the victimisation began. The shame then the blame, then the anger and back to feeling ashamed; around and around. I had no one else to blame but myself. I was so out of kilter that not only did I yearn to have

Scott call me to apologise (which he never would), I also needed to have him acknowledge me. It never eventuated.

When Mum asked about my day prior, I told her we'd broken up.

'Oh, that's why you look terrible this morning. You'll be fine, put it behind you and move on. I didn't like him anyway.'

Having your mother tell you that always makes you feel better, right? No, she didn't know a quarter of what I put myself through. I internalised everything to the most minute detail, replaying the gun incident and all others that came before it. My mind repeated the incident continually over and over during the following weeks. My anxiousness caused me to stop eating and my weight dropped to a dangerous level for my height. I'm only 167 centimetres and I got down to 42 kilograms. I was nothing but skin on bone.

Mum witnessed me leaving the shower and heading to my bedroom one night without a towel around me as I thought she'd gone to bed. She dropped the glass she was holding, shocked by my skeletal frame. My parents then berated me for thinking I was making myself ill because I was trying to lose weight to look good. Dad would yell at me at the dinner table.

'Who would want to be with you? You look disgusting.' He'd get up and leave.

At times I'd swallow food to pacify them, only to crouch at the toilet and vomit when dinner was over. I didn't need to stick my fingers down my throat to purge, I just thought about what had taken place weeks earlier and it would happen automatically.

I developed ulcerative colitis, an illness that still raises its head today if I get too stressed. My lower bowel lining bleeds and the pain is indescribable. My nervous system also shuts down, so if get over-tired I will spend days in bed recovering. I had large cold sores appear on my lips and aching ulcers in my mouth, I'd wake up with blood in my pillow. Then I contracted shingles. I was a complete mess, physically, mentally and emotionally.

All the effort Mum put in nursing me back to health over an eight-week period in my mind was still no use. Everyone was just going about their lives as normal but I had finally hit rock bottom again. It was then that I decided that I couldn't go on any longer. It had to stop. I was going to take my life.

2002

Reaching a point where I felt I had to end the madness that kept going around my mind almost gave me relief, but then I experienced another manic episode. It was purely fight or flight. It was triggered from deciding to take my life. The switch occurred very quickly but then in a concession of extremes: pure blackness and depth then shining euphoria. I was going to commit suicide but I felt so strongly that I needed to achieve something significant prior to leaving to prove I wasn't a complete failure. I wanted to be remembered for having made something good of my life before I took it.

My answer: landing an incredible job in real estate marketing.

Let me put this in perspective for you. I'd never studied marketing, let alone had any knowledge of real estate, but my manic enthusiasm zoned in and worked its magic. After two interviews over as many days I was starting a new job on the coming Monday. That's when I went into a complete mental tailspin that only I noticed as I had the 'perfect mask' on again. It was pure panic and anxiety rushing through me. My family were ecstatic though. To them I'd come out of an extremely dark period and gotten through to the other side, the sunny side of hell. I hadn't though; it was an illusion.

A few months prior I had a gun pointed at my head, which I hadn't been able to process, then I gained an extremely high-pressure job with a company in a field I had no experience in. I was a complete fraud and within my mind no other option was plausible. I was disgusted in myself and started trying to work out how to end my life.

One day, Dad decided to go into the MCG and see a game. Knowing I'd made an effort to go out and get a new job, he invited me along but I politely declined telling him that I wanted to rest up before Monday. As soon as he left the house, I dropped into automatic. I drove down to the hardware store and bought a container of Stanley knife blades, then headed back. With a full container of prescribed sleeping medication, I swallowed them down with whisky and began writing a note apologising to my family for being such an utter, complete failure.

I'd thought about driving to nearby bushland and carrying out my plan somewhere secluded but then thought that if Mum and my sisters didn't have a body to bury it'd be worse for them. Getting out of the car I then headed to my bed, and started slicing at my wrists. There was an old black and white photo by my bedside that I noticed; it was of me sitting on Mum's knee when I was one, surrounded by my sisters. I was smiling back at myself. Who'd have known then that such a cute little kid would become a complete fuckup. I despised myself that much.

I know I didn't choose suicide for attention. Who the hell wants attention when they are so out of their mind with severe manic episodes that they stand out like a golden child full of electricity one minute, only to collapse into a complete disaster, bouncing from one catastrophe to another, feeling ashamed and defective? I wanted out. I needed the grief I felt day and night, nonstop, to end. The extreme peaks and the darkest of holes, that's what I existed on, unless I was medicated and then I'd become a pharmaceutical zombie. I needed it to cease. I was beyond tired.

I considered what my family and friends would say.

'How could you? How could you be so selfish?'

That to me was easy to answer. I wasn't a parent. I wasn't married. I didn't have a partner. I didn't have anyone dependent on me. I was someone's daughter. I was one of four kids, the youngest, and I felt like a burden; it was a guilt-free ticket out. So why wouldn't I? And how dare anyone shame me when they didn't experience the relentless noise that was constantly on repeat in my mind.

Feeling tired and cold I prayed that the pain I felt in my chest and the chatter in my head would soon end. I wanted to feel nothing. I then drifted off into blackness.

Next thing I felt was a jolt of light, then a sharp pain in my head as Mum pushed me into the back of her car. I could hear her muffled shouting at Dad. I blacked out again. A dream of being laid out, floating and bumping, lots of bumping, a feeling of falling, but I didn't land anywhere, instead I spun, to one side then the other. My throat hurt.

Then I woke up. I was flat, lying on a hospital trolley, my whole family surrounding me. Their faces were ashen; they looked horrified, just staring at me. Mum's shirt had blood on it. Dad. Jane and Anne alongside their husbands. I had been given charcoal via a tube down my throat. Again, I'd failed, tears streaking my face. My newly wound bandages on my arms. Why did they wake me? I was so angry, drugged and angry.

'I can't believe you did that. You weren't meant to do that. I'm not meant to be here. I'm in the wrong place.' I was furious. I passed out again.

It was only from my mother's instincts that Dad hadn't seen me for a few hours that something triggered her to go straight into my room. Registering the bottle of pills and blades on my bed sheets she grabbed me, screaming at Dad to get the car. She didn't even think of calling an ambulance. Dad sped to the hospital's emergency room with Mum in the back of the car shaking me to wake up. Emergency staff pulled me out of the car, knocking the side of my head in the process, and threw me on a gurney.

I was not at peace with being saved at the time though. I was not grateful. Anne slept by my bedside every night in hospital. I had a nurse during the day as I was on suicide watch. It was Mum's decision not to have me committed to the psychiatric ward. She explained that she felt so incredibly guilty for not getting to me sooner, for not understanding how ill I was. But it wasn't her fault – no one was to know.

Once I'd been discharged, we headed back home only to have to stop to pick some bread up at the supermarket. Mum wanted me to go with her and as we reached the cashier with a loaf of Tip Top in our possession, the lady at the cash register noticed I still had my hospital ID bracelet on. She was super cheery.

'Oh, wow you've just gotten out of hospital. Your wrist is bandaged. I hope you're OK? What were you in for?'

Mum braced for the answer to the question, knowing full well sometimes I didn't have a filter when I was tired. And she was right. I was drained and, completely straight-faced, almost deadpan, said, 'I tried to kill myself last week.'

The poor woman's mouth dropped open and she didn't know what to say. Mum sighed heavily out of exhaustion, apologised and we calmly collected our purchase and walked back to the car.

I have felt the grief others feel for losing their loved ones to suicide. I have seen the agonising bereavement that leeches through those remaining, replaced by enormous anger, then emptiness, only to then repeat.

'I don't understand, it makes no sense. Why didn't you say something?'

That's the blame.

'I should have known.'

That's the guilt.

'You're so selfish. Do you know what you nearly did?'

That's the anger.

'Why?'

So many questions, thinking you know the answer. You don't.

I was to understand everything that my family was left to feel much later. They got to peer into what it could have been like, being left behind to deal with the enormous loss, an endless hole that can't be filled. Parents who could have lost a child. Siblings and friends so angry and horrified. What could have been tragic, beyond understanding.

From their perspective when they last saw me, I had seemed fine. I'd been on the road to recovery. I was getting better. They'd witnessed me laughing and chatting with what seemed like not a care in the world but what they didn't understand was how someone who wants to take their life will play any role to remain undetected. I wanted to step out of life with a silent movement. Nothing was logical. More nights than not I would put my head on my pillow and on rotation the voices would overshadow everything positive that may have occurred. The mental pain was all-consuming – I'd started to drown in it. I was nearly fully immersed and I didn't have the strength to hold my head above water anymore.

Once at home I was horrified when I found out that Dad had called the director of the estate agency to explain that I wasn't going to be taking up the position. I grabbed my phone and ran to my bedroom, putting on that happy mask, and called the company personally to tell them there had been a mistake. I was ready to start that afternoon, but it fell on deaf ears. The receptionist was almost embarrassed by my call.

'I'm sorry, Jackie, the role has been passed to another candidate. Take care.'

The line then went dead.

I was back where I'd started, with an enormous ache in my heart and a voice in my head that just wouldn't go away. It was deafening; I was lost. What I hadn't seen that was so obviously in front of me was that I was responsible for not moving forward, but I also understand now that I was extremely unwell and needed further medical treatment.

Next move: my manic thought process moved into top gear knowing that if I was spared my life then I would have to try even harder than before to do the right thing by others, as though I didn't try hard enough last time. If I was kind then I would be shown kindness in return. Only then I would be treated well. And there lay the next mistake. It was repetitious. Again, I saw other people saving me from myself.

Even stronger than before, I needed someone who knew better than I did and would guide me through life: a teacher of sorts. I made the decision to officially be baptised at the church I'd been attending. In my mind this was a fresh start. I asked Clair's husband William if he would do the honours. I stood in the baptism bath one Sunday night and he placed his hand gently on my forehead as he spoke the words that I felt would change me from being an enormous failure to someone who would have a second chance at making everything right in my life. My parents didn't attend but they supported me in anything that would have a positive influence.

As my health slowly improved over a few months, I decided I wanted to leave their house and start anew. They would only let me leave if I had somewhere they considered safe, so Clair's parents had offered me a room within their own home just outside of Melbourne. I decided to take up the opportunity to live in the Yarra Valley for a while until I was strong enough to look for work again.

It was the simple act of Clair's parents' support that helped strengthen my soul and eventually returned my physical health. Theirs was a nurturing environment where I was never on high alert as they weren't drinkers. Everything was always calmly discussed with a dash of humour to keep the endorphins flowing, rather than turning into an alcohol-fuelled explosion, one where you knew it wouldn't end well no matter how hard you tried to steer it. To be in Clair's father's company taught me that there were positive male role models. This was due not only to his wise attributes but from watching Harry since I was a young girl raising Clair along with her mum, Eve, and how they treated her with such respect. Unfortunately, over time the warmth and comfort I felt within their home didn't supress how uncomfortable I could be with my own company.

Within a couple of months my life started again to pivot on the wish for a man in my life and my self-professed theory that once I was married everything would be perfect. I yearned to be wanted and to be needed; it was like I was missing a drug that I was dependent on, but I wouldn't go out to get a quick fix. I wanted a solid commitment.

Enter the man who was to become my second husband: David. David wasn't a church member, more a disgruntled ex-Catholic.

I was still at church when we met but it didn't take long for panic to set in again as I felt I was living two very different lives. One where I was who I wanted to be, a good Christian, and the other one, where I needed and wanted a man in my life, thinking it would make everything better. I wasn't willing to believe or even confront that neither was the answer.

One Sunday morning, as I sat in a pew at church, the bishop began his sermon. The lesson was based on honesty. I started to feel an anxious state about the life I was leading. I could see how hypocritical I was in the way I was living and I couldn't do it anymore. I stood up and walked out. I left the church feeling that I was a complete fraud and never returned. It wasn't enough that I had let myself down but I felt I let Clair and her family down. I was overcome again by shame.

I see my time with David as receiving the mother lode of all lessons as I still hadn't learned or understood I was purely responsible for my life. I was still hanging on to the idea that someone out there was going to save and help me become a better person, one that would be perfectly perfect.

2004

David and I met on a new website set up for singles who wanted to meet with the hope of starting a relationship. I was so happy when, after only having my profile online for just over a day, I received a 'kiss' from a guy who used the pseudonym 777Ben. My friends were coaching me on the etiquette of being online and laid out some rules:

1. Really get to know the person before meeting up.

2. Don't rush meeting up in person, take your time.

3. If you do meet up start with something simple like a coffee just to gauge the person.

4. Let someone know where you're going and the time you'll be on your date.

5. Never meet up somewhere dark and dingy.

And finally:
- Never get into their car.

Armed with all this wonderful information to tackle the new world of online dating, I went forth, and without even trying to I broke every single rule!

The first time we met up after only after a couple of messages and David seemed very shy. He kept his head down and didn't look at me directly in the eyes, which is something that's always been a pet peeve of mine. The conversation warmed as the evening went on. We were only meant to meet up for a few hours over dinner but it turned into nine hours with me being driven all over Melbourne in his car to different restaurants and cafés.

David was in the hospitality industry and his persona brightened as the evening went on, as he seemed to know everyone. We laughed, talked and had a wonderful night, which ended with me not getting home until 4 am. I was dizzy with happiness and the following day David texted me to say he had a wonderful evening.

We exchanged in-depth emails until we met up the following Saturday night. Again, we went to a restaurant in the city that I chose, but after the meal he told me he was unimpressed. Not wanting to see him upset, I told him I'd foot the bill.

After we finished, we drove home to his sister's house where he said he paid half the mortgage to help her out since he'd sold his own home earlier that year. As we sat out the front to say our goodbyes, David looked disappointed. He told me that his sister had asked him not to come home that night as she was having her boyfriend over so he told me that he didn't have anywhere to sleep. He was going to head over to his place of business and sleep out the back on a sofa. Being Miss Fix-it, I immediately told him that there was a spare bed at my place so he could stay, as I felt sorry for him. When we got there he gazed around wide-eyed telling me what an amazing house I had, joking that I must be very wealthy. I laughed and told him I was housesitting my parents place as I did every winter when they headed up north to escape the cold. As he looked around he noticed the bar and informed me that he loved port. I immediately poured him a glass and got the fireplace going to help warm us up.

I didn't drink that night, as I couldn't stand port. As soon as I showed David the spare room he turned around and kissed me, saying that he'd prefer to sleep in my bed. I hesitated in that split second but then thought, as we were both adults, why not.

The following morning my brother-in-law Andrew turned up at the house for something in Dad's garage. No sooner had I stepped outside to greet him when David rushed past us just as Andrew put his hand out to introduce himself. He got into his car and took off. I put it down to him being shy, as I was good at seeing everything through rose-coloured glasses. Andrew wasn't impressed; I could see it written over his face.

Not only would David text me three or four times a night while he was working, but there were times I'd wake in the morning and head to my car to find he'd driven half an hour to where I lived and placed a love note under my windscreen wiper. Some would see it as a bit full on. I was completely smitten.

On show from the very beginning were our differences. My new outlook on the world – a sunny and kind disposition – matched him, as he was controlled, street smart and very clever. I found it refreshing. He said I needed to toughen up and stand on my own two feet away from my family and friends and he was the one who was going to help me. I felt grateful that he would take the time to do that.

'Jackie, when the student is ready the teacher will come.'

He was definitely in charge and that was music to my ears.

In my eyes it was pure blossoming love. After eight weeks of dating, I arrived at work one morning to read an email from him telling me that he had something he needed to speak with me about. I went into an immediate meltdown thinking that he wanted to break up. Instead he wrote telling me that he wasn't the age that I'd been led to believe over the last eight weeks. He was actually forty, not thirty-two, as he'd told me. Instead of questioning why he lied to me, I was incredibly relieved that he didn't want to split up.

The following day was a Saturday and we spent it in bed, only leaving our cocoon to get Chinese for lunch. Once we returned to bed with our meal of fried rice and Mongolian beef, just before we broke a bar of chocolate for dessert, he asked me to marry him. He said that he wanted us to elope overseas – that way it would just be the two of us. It was the 'us against the world' mentality that I interpreted as romantic. I felt so special as he only wanted me. I was immersed in pure bliss knowing that someone actually wanted to marry me again. He was devoted to me and I him.

Apart from running past Andrew eight weeks prior, he'd never met any of my family or friends. He'd always been too busy.

The following day I jogged over to Clair's house to tell her the good news. She could see that I was elated beyond comprehension and it scared the living daylights out of her. Clair was never backwards in telling me how she felt, which is why I loved her but her response to my news left me gutted. She was the voice of reason and I didn't want to hear anything she had to say so I left her house. Once home I called David to tell him how crushed I was by her reaction.

'She's just jealous, Jack, and now more than ever you don't need this. It's time you started shedding these negative influences in your life or you'll never be able to move forward, or maybe you don't want to. Maybe you want to surround yourself in people who wish to hold you back? It's your choice.' He hung up.

I was left sitting with a huge sense of guilt. Within hours that guilt turned into anger because I was feeling threatened. No one was going to take away what I perceived to be my ultimate goal. I needed to prove how dedicated I was to this man I loved.

Clair called and asked me to dinner the following week. We scooted around the elephant in the room but when the evening ended she spoke about what had transpired seven days previously. As any best friend would, she offered up words of concern around my behaviour since David had arrived on the scene.

Instead of listening, my reaction was to sit with a huge amount of hurt, insulted that she spoke of him with such disregard. In hindsight I was never going to listen to what she had to say anyway. I then mentally proceeded to blow everything out of proportion, as I needed any viable excuse to cut ties. I wanted to prove to David that he could trust me to support him. I walked away barley having said a word to Clair, the conversations were only in my head.

The following day David told me the best thing I could do was write her a letter and tell her our friendship was over. I did as he advised. When I saw her number come up on my phone, I ignored it to the point where Clair left a message telling me I was a coward for not speaking to her. I put it down to David's theory of jealousy and left it at that. And that is how you break an unbreakable friendship with your best friend – simple.

Jane was ropable when she found out that I'd chosen this bloke no one knew over my best friend who'd I'd known since

I was fourteen. I was so blinded by what was in front of me but I didn't want to hear what anyone had to say. I stopped seeing my family as often as I had in the past. David told me that it was best, as they didn't understand us.

When my parents returned home from their holiday, I started to look for a new apartment to rent. As soon as I found one David said he wanted to accompany me to see that I'd chosen the right place. Lately he had insisted on looking over a lot my choices, saying that because he was older than me it was best. Again, I agreed because it made me feel special that someone wanted to look out for me.

Just as I was about to sign a lease agreement, he told me he wanted me to move into the place he shared with his sister, Melissa. He said he'd been thinking about it for a while and he'd spoken to her, as he couldn't wait for us to marry to start our new life together. Melissa wanted me to pay 250 dollars a week and I was to do all the housework. It used to be David's job but he was working a lot and didn't have the time. I happily agreed.

On my thirty-fifth birthday, just before I moved in, Mum said it was time that she and Dad meet the man I was engaged to. David turned up to take me to dinner with a beautiful bunch of flowers and a disc of music he liked that he'd made up for me. When Mum asked him if the flowers were from a florist she knew had a good reputation, he looked at her with a straight face.

'God, no. She's not worth that much.'

Funnily enough, my father had said the same thing about me when I was in hospital as a teenager. It stung just as much but I ignored it.

We went to dinner at a restaurant I wanted to try and after we'd returned to the car David started berating me that it was the worst meal that he'd ever had and it was my fault for thinking I could choose a place as I didn't know a thing about food. I was hurt and embarrassed but even though it was my birthday I gave him the money that it cost him. Anything to calm him down.

No sooner had I moved in with him when major changes started to happen. On the first day he wouldn't speak to me and left for work. He didn't come home that night and I was so worried that I tried to call and text him but his phone was off. When he walked in twenty-four hours later, he looked at me like I was crazy for asking where he was. He then took me into his arms and told me everything was all right, but I had to toughen up, as there'd be nights that he wouldn't come home. This was news to me. It made me see how desperate I was but I tried to brush it off as me being silly. I didn't want to cause a scene.

We'd been engaged for a month but still David hadn't yet bought me a ring. Melissa insisted that he buy me one immediately. I told her I wasn't into jewellery. She looked horrified, obviously seeing it as a lack of self-worth.

'Oh my God, I know David's tight but he's not getting away with this. It's only proper that he buys you a ring to prove to you how much he loves you. You're worth a ring, Jackie.'

I had no expectation of what I deserved in life so it was Melissa who helped me design a ring and decide what stones went into it. I was happy with simple gems but she wouldn't have any of it because she knew David could afford a five-carat diamond. I settled for a tiny diamond accompanied by our birthstones, as we were born in the same month.

One night when David was at work and I'd gone to bed early, there was a knock on my door. It was Melissa – she wanted to speak to me. I got out of bed and followed her into the lounge room. She'd been drinking; there was such disdain in her voice.

'Why did you move into my house without asking me first? Do you think doing house work every week should be considered payment enough to live under my roof?'

I couldn't understand what she was talking about and I must have looked completely baffled and bewildered, so she started to spell it out.

'You are living under my roof. David stupidly sold his home, made a huge profit – it was a cash sale. He's since moved into my home as I offered him a place to stay for a few weeks. That was six months ago. He's never paid me rent, stashing his money away like a squirrel planning for winter.'

'Melissa, I've been paying you rent. 250 dollars a week.

It then hit me square in the face what was happening. I was paying David 250 dollars a week, but she'd never seen any of it. She was also sick to death of paying for all the food we consumed. To say I was left embarrassed and numb was an understatement, but I thought David would have an explanation.

She looked at me in disgust, telling me that if I was that stupid, I deserved everything her brother dished out. 'Kid, you're swimming with a shark, the "black sheep" of our family, the "dark horse" – name it what you will. I have no idea how to make it any clearer for you. You'd better wake up and deal with it or run.'

I didn't run. I just went to bed and cried myself to sleep.

When David finally returned home in the wee hours of the following morning, I burst into tears again and told him what happened. He was fuming and told me that Melissa was a bitch. He said she'd fabricated the whole thing, so we moved out the following week having found a place to rent. He paid the bond. He then said he hadn't budgeted for the mess I'd caused with his sister, which cost him over 3000 dollars, and that I owed him. I never questioned it, as I felt completely guilty about everything that was happening around me.

Seven months after our engagement, we sat at Tullamarine airport waiting for our flight to take us to New Zealand's South Island where we'd organised for our wedding to be held. I had a glimpse of regret that none of my family were going to be present to witness the event, even though Anne begged me to stay in Australia because she was worried about what I was getting myself into. My family saw all the red flags. I, on the other hand, ignored them, making excuses for his behaviour.

We were a week into our month-long trip and we were sitting at a bar before we went to see a movie. It dawned on me; for all the time that we'd been together we'd never gone out to something as simple as the cinema. All I'd ever done was wait at home for him, never ventured out and enjoyed myself with friends because I felt guilty that he was working, even though I too was holding down a full-time job during the day. David could obviously see the distress on my face. I told him that I'd already been a part of one failed marriage and I didn't want another so I was having second thoughts. It was something so simple but it was as though my eyes were now wide open. He went into overdrive, telling me that I was being unreasonable, that he'd been working hard to save for our future together and I was being selfish.

Just as I went to get up and walk off, his eyes filled with tears and he told me that if we didn't marry his family would see him as a laughing stock. I was that quickly turned, a moment of clarity snuffed. We went to the movies and he was so tactile, kissing and hugging me until I forgot my worries. When we returned to the hotel he made love to me like he'd never done before. He was so tender and caring; all was forgiven and forgotten.

The following week was our wedding day and it was a day of 'red flags', so many it could have been used as bunting for our big day. I left our hotel after lunch to have my hair and makeup done. When I arrived back at our room, we dressed and as we were waiting in the lobby for the car to take us to the chapel at sunset David decided to throw a diva tantrum, that which I'd never witnessed before. Behaving like a complete irrational child he started.

'Oh my God, why isn't anyone looking at me? Why is everyone saying you look amazing and not me?'

Completely speechless, again I ignored his behaviour.

When we finally arrived at our destination, David immediately headed for Sandy, a photographer who he'd booked online. The wedding celebrant had to pull him away from chatting to her so the ceremony could begin.

After the formalities were over, we were left on the beach to share a picnic basket near where our ceremony had taken place. David told me he had a brilliant idea. I was waiting for him to tell me he had arranged something special, as the evening was young.

'Let's go to a restaurant in Arrowtown where Sandy told me she's gone on a date and we can join her!'

'David, it's our wedding night. Let's do something together.'

'Fuck, Jack, you're already sounding like a nagging wife. Get over it.'

Stunned, I shut my mouth and got in the car.

We arrived just as Sandy and her date were being served dessert, so David ordered for us and Sandy took some pictures of him feeding me apple pie and ice cream. When she headed over to the bar, David got up and followed her. I was waiting at the table with Sandy's date. I looked over and she was leaning up against the bar. David had his hand resting on her ass. I froze with astonishment. I didn't know where to turn. Sandy's date turned to look in the same direction then went over to the bar. He had a word to the two of them then left the restaurant, slamming the door behind him. Sandy ran after the guy and David continued drinking by himself, as if nothing happened. Only hours previously I'd wed this man and he'd just physically made a move on the photographer. I was left sitting at the table, too embarrassed to move. All that came to mind was Mum always telling me not to make a scene in public. Believe me, when you're sitting in a public place wearing a bridal gown people do not look in the other direction. I had middle-aged women who'd had too much to drink swamping me from every direction, telling me that they wanted to catch my bouquet! I can laugh at it now but it was incredibly humiliating at the time. I didn't act on my instinct.

We returned to our suite and I was so angry I couldn't even look at him. He told me he had a headache and wanted to sleep, which I was more than happy about. He didn't touch me for the following three nights and instead of being gutted I wish I had the foresight to annul the marriage due to having not consummated it.

When he went to bed, I stayed up holding the faxes that had been sent by my family wishing us happiness for the rest of our lives together. What they would never know was that it hadn't gotten off to a great start. But then I did exactly what Mum would have been proud of: I held my head high, as it's what would have been expected for any woman in our family. I got on with the remainder of our honeymoon, putting it behind me.

If I'd called home to Australia and explained the situation, I have no doubt in my mind that my sisters would have jumped into action and done all they could to have gotten me on the next plane out of there. But that would have been another failure. I felt I had no one to turn to.

And so married life began.

2005

Once we returned home from overseas, I decided that I was going to do everything possible to make the marriage work no matter what. I'd even placed Louise Hay's affirmation cards on the fridge that stated: 'I am in a joyous, intimate relationship with a person who truly loves me' and 'My partner is the love of my life. We adore each other'. Pity they didn't come with a money-back guarantee – not that it was Louise Hay's fault, may she rest in peace. I know she had the best of intentions at heart when she envisioned the colourful and glossy double-sided cardboard. What I didn't realise was that it takes both parties in a marriage to make it work.

On our return from our trip, we hosted a small wedding reception at a hotel in the city. After our family had dined and tried their hardest to congratulate us, David decided he'd wouldn't speak to me. For what reason, I was never to know. Once at home and I was out of the car, he took off. I didn't see him for twenty-four hours. I took it all on my shoulders as my fault but I didn't understand why. I never discussed it with anyone – I felt embarrassed as it reflected badly on me as a wife. I was someone who couldn't keep her husband happy.

It became a near daily event where nothing was ever good enough or he'd taunt me about the most ridiculous things. Whatever I said he would reply in the negative and add that I was either stupid, ignorant or both. To him my job never brought in enough money for his liking so I went out to find something else to do that he approved of. I was never allowed to see anything financial, though, as he told me I was too stupid to understand it and I wasn't worthy of knowing such information. All I had to do was work, placing all my earnings into paying for the mortgage.

One afternoon I jokingly mentioned that I knew where he stashed all his spare cash. He swung around and grabbed me tightly around my wrist then twisted it behind my back, telling me if I ever mentioned it to anyone and the word got out to the ATO I'd be going to jail alongside him.

He started withholding sex from me after we married. He knew I'd enjoyed a healthy sexual relationship in the past and he started using it against me as a control tool. No matter what I said, how I looked or what I wore to bed nothing would coerce him into sex.

I felt so humiliated. My girlfriends were always complaining that their husbands wouldn't stop touching them and they envied me. To go from someone who had a partner who wanted sex to then have nothing made me feel like a desperate freak. It shamed me terribly when he eventually told me I repulsed him. I'd gone out especially and bought a pretty nightie. It was debilitating and all I ever asked myself was the same thing I always did: *What's wrong with me?* He would just look me up and down, shaking his head in disbelief as though I was too stupid to see it myself and roll over. I felt absolutely gutted and I couldn't win; the silence was worse than having an argument.

He often spoke about other women he met whilst single and his sexual encounters, but I never saw any evidence that he was interested in me at all. He was emotionally and sexually disconnected. If he ever woke me when he came to bed at three in the morning it was never for sex – he did it to start fights, but they were pretty much one-sided as he'd bait me, wind me up then turn over and fall asleep leaving me wide awake. It nearly sent me crazy. I would lose that much sleep that I'd end up in tears from exhaustion unable to function the following day. Another trait was his perpetual and unconventional behaviour. I have a feeling David helped coin the international phrase 'gaslighting'.

Dad had handmade all his children an outdoor lounge seat and it was special to me. One day after David returned from a run, he was doing his cooling down exercises and started doing jumps, landing his weight on and off the chair. Well, it didn't take long before the chair broke in two, collapsing under his weight. But when I angrily approached him, instead of apologising, he swore that he didn't do it.

'It's a shit piece of furniture that just collapsed. Fucking get over it.'

If any of my family invited us around for dinner he'd purposely start a fight over nothing about an hour before we were to leave. I'd be so upset I couldn't go out or he'd refuse to come so I went to a lot of family gatherings on my own. It was better that way anyway because, if he did come, he'd just insult my family when we returned to the car.

If I'd invited others over he'd start yelling at me that he hated people invading his private space. When they arrived I'd be all red-faced and puffy-eyed from crying. He'd behave as if nothing was wrong.

We did invite one of his employees over one night, Jake, and his wife, Kaitlin, which turned out to be one of the most bizarre dinners I've ever hosted. David sat opposite Jake and chatted to him all night, completely ignoring Kaitlin and me to the point of embarrassment. If we attempted to join in the conversation David would dismiss everything we said with a raising of his hand. I had never been in a position like that and it was completely unsettling to witness. David was literally giggling with Jake at everything he said and it wasn't even funny banter. I wasn't only uncomfortable watching his behaviour but it was as though Kaitlin and I weren't at all present at the table and David was on a first date.

It wasn't too long after that night when I came across pictures and videos he had on his computer depicting women and men of all ages in pornographic images. I also came across other sites with correspondence to and from women and men from all over Australia. OK, when I say I 'came across' them I mean that I couldn't stop hearing my inner voice telling me something was truly off. While he was at work late one afternoon, I went into our study and went to his laptop. I morphed into Dora The Explorer. And there it was: the dates of the correspondence coincided with the time we started dating and after we had married. There was a video that was so disturbing but also confusing at the same time. The female in it had to be underage, maybe fifteen, which was bad enough but she was surrounded by seven naked men.

As the image played out in front of me, it was appalling the way the young girl was treated.

I went to sleep with questions spinning around my mind but prepared to speak with him about it, as I needed answers. I'd had it with this marriage, this man I didn't know. I was over the charade and wanted out.

The following afternoon, before David went to work, I approached him. I calmly told him what I'd found on the computer. By this stage I was feeling completely confused because of all the effort I'd made to try and make this sham of a marriage work. I started telling him that I thought he was a hypocrite for always taking the high moral ground over me when I'd seen the messages and the girl in the video.

He then said something that I never saw coming. 'The girl in the video isn't what I'm interested in.'

My voice started rising out of anger. 'What are you talking about? It's there. I've seen it.'

With his head tilted and a look on his face that was blank he spoke. 'I like watching the men. I'm into men.'

I stood, stunned but silent, staring at him with the words echoing in my mind. I was numb. Leaning forward as though I hadn't heard correctly, I said, 'You're interested in the men, not the girl?'

He nodded. 'Yes.' He confirmed it.

I must have looked like I'd been struck with a rod. My mouth was open and my eyes were wide.

He then slowly turned towards the door, picked up his satchel, closed the door behind himself and drove off.

I felt numb. To start with, all I could think about was how I could help him change his mind, which was such an ego-driven thought – I just couldn't take the rejection. I was married to a man who wanted to be with other guys. After sitting with it for a few hours, I decided to do the right thing and leave the marriage. To begin with I felt angry but eventually that lessened and empathy took its place.

After he returned from work that night, he didn't speak to me for three days straight. I couldn't even get him to respond to the slightest of exchanges. He gave me the silent treatment, turning the table on me to make me think I had done the wrong thing. Had I? I was never one to judge someone's sexuality but if you're married and there's been no discussion about having an open marriage with either sex, how can that be fair? I couldn't live in an open marriage, now or ever, so was that fair on his behalf? I went from feeling compassion for the situation he was in to feeling guilty, which stopped me from leaving. I turned it into being my fault because ultimately I shouldn't have been snooping around his computer.

Psychologically things became almost unbearable. At home he treated me like I didn't exist. I cooked him dinner every night and had it waiting for him when he got home. He'd pick up the plate and scrape it into the rubbish. But if I didn't cook for him, he'd be furious. I was so confused because in public he treated me like a queen. After we'd get home, he'd start a fight. I'd be in tears. He'd attempt to soothe me then he'd want sex, but it wasn't caring and loving – there was never any emotion. It was crazy behaviour to live with, and exhausting never knowing his mood. We never broached the subject again though – it was buried.

It was then I decided to approach a marriage counsellor to see what I could do to make it better. I was brought up that it was a woman's duty to keep the man of the household happy. After I disclosed to the therapist what I had been putting up with, she pointed out the warning signs for me to go over. She encouraged me to make a decision about leaving the marriage.

'Jackie, I would strongly recommend to plan how and when you're going to leave. Explain what's going on to your closest friends or family. You'll need them for support.'

Fate came along, though, and played a card that changed the plan of leaving. Through that miraculous event of marital intercourse, I had fallen pregnant.

2006

I was shocked but then elated. I'd so wanted a child because I was not getting any younger at thirty-six. The maternal Big Ben had been ticking away in my subconscious. I was desperate to be a mother. Even though I was planning to leave the marriage, it was as if this pregnancy, this child, brought new hope. David and I were not in sync. I thought that maybe once we were but that was a dream; we never were, never would be, and not even a child was going to fix that.

After conducting two home pregnancy tests, I approached David. He was in the bathroom shaving. I told him I had some wonderful news and foolishly thought it would be a new beginning for us. Keep in mind, I'd suffered four miscarriages in the past, so having a child was a dream I truly hoped would happen but thought it just wouldn't.

'David, we're going to have a baby.'

His face went blank and all he could say after what would be considered an uncomfortable silence was the following.

'Congratulations, Jackie ... good for you.'

He raised his eyebrows and, in a swift moment, he said, 'Did I ever tell you that I made two of my past girlfriends have an abortion?'

It was from that night on I knew it was inevitable, so I started thinking along the lines of a single parent; just the baby and I. My instinct told me I was going to have a little boy. Every moment was spent thinking positive things for my baby, singing to him and eating the correct foods and feeling that I was solely responsible for bringing this child into the world. At twelve weeks pregnant I developed pneumonia and had to drive myself to the hospital as David said he was too busy. At six months I was so tired one morning on the way to work I ran my car into the back of a truck. I was so upset as to what David would say about me crashing my car so I ignored the paramedic who'd been called got a taxi home. After waking David to explain what had happened, I started to feel the impact of the crash. Knowing I had to check the baby was all right, I drove David's car to the hospital for tests as he refused to get out of bed. He'd told me to have his car back by the time he had to go to work, then turned over and resumed his sleep.

One morning at twenty weeks, he came into the kitchen, screaming at me.

'What impact do you think this fuckup will have on my life? You never considered how it would impact me. You're a fucking selfish bitch.'

Cowering, I braced myself for the impact. Finally, he walked away, bewildered and shocked by the words he bestowed on his pregnant wife.

After nine months of dealing with David only doting on me in public, acting the excited expectant father-to-be and then in private yelling continually as his personal diva emerged again and again from its cocoon, our son finally arrived after twenty-eight hours of labour at our local hospital. With only a midwife and David present during the natural birth, all I can say is that it had the most incredibly positive impact on me, which I believe influenced my new direction. My view on life from that day on was this: I was officially ready to step up and take responsibility for my life. The reason being that if I, as a woman, could endure pregnancy for nine months then labour as well as the actual birth, then I could do anything. Nothing could stop me and that wasn't a delusional manic thought; it was the most rational one I have ever had in my life to date. It was then I officially removed David from the pedestal I'd originally put him on.

David never contacted my family to inform them of our healthy and beautiful son's arrival until two days after the event occurred. He told me that he'd notified them but they were too busy to come to the hospital.

Whilst I was in the final stages of labour at home, he'd contacted my sister Jane when she was at work and told her she needed her to come over to our house because he had to go to work.

'David, I don't know if you know this but it's your job as Jack's husband to stay with her so step up,' Jane told him.

He never forgave her and he turned what should have been a family celebration into a game, so my family missed out on seeing its newest member.

I was in hospital for five days after the birth. On the day I was to head home with Angus, David told me he had to go interstate on business so he wouldn't return until the following evening. I didn't have any money to buy all the basics a parent would purchase to fill their new child's nursery with and I was too proud to ask my family for help. Before I left the hospital, I stole a single bed sheet and, once Anne had dropped me at home and left me alone, I pulled it out of my small suitcase and cut it into four makeshift cot sheets.

Four weeks later I returned to the hospital's administration building and, having asked Mum for a loan of fifty dollars, I made a donation to cover my theft. I felt so guilty. The smiling receptionist was elated.

'Thank you, that's so kind. Can I have your name and number for our record?'

'Ah no, thanks for asking but I want it to be anonymous.' Spoken like I was a true philanthropist. Yeah, more like I was so horrified by my behaviour that I didn't want the police knocking on my door because the linen management department had noticed that their bed sheet count was incorrect and they'd tracked me down. I wish she'd just angrily stared at me, pointed her finger directly at me, knowing the shame I felt.

'So you're the sheet stealer we've been looking for? Shame on you! Don't move – I'm calling the cops.'

Once David arrived home the following day, he did and said things that astounded me. The house was too messy for his liking and dinner needed to be on the table even though he'd decided my cooking was crap. As I wasn't working and bringing any money into the house it was official: I was 'sponging' off him. The outside temperature was hitting forty-five degrees that summer and David insisted that I go out food shopping. I had given birth less than seven days prior so I was still bleeding heavily and physically exhausted. It wore me down terribly. I started drinking again as David worked until late.

David's mother knew I didn't have any money of my own so she started giving me one hundred dollars a week that I had to keep secret. She knew his nature and his ability to be selfish. At least I had something to buy formula and nappies for Angus.

Anything could set David off and he was always looking for a reason to yell. I told him only what he wanted to hear – I never spoke my mind. When the federal government kindly decided to give us over three thousand dollars as a baby bonus, David went out and bought a John Deer ride-on mower so it didn't take him as long to mow our lawn.

I was so grateful that Angus was such a happy baby and a good sleeper too, but as soon as I put him to bed at night, I could take off my 'perfectly happy mummy' mask and then I was left facing the stark reality of what a mess my marriage was and what type of home I'd be raising him in. Getting dinner ready became even more problematic as I would stare at the sharp knives I was using to cut up the vegetables. I would visualise running the blade up my arm time and again.

When David got home, it would be his turn to feed his son via a bottle, as Angus wouldn't latch on to my breast. David ticked that off as another fault of mine too. When I heard his car coming down the driveway and I was still up I'd run to our bedroom, jump into bed and pretend to be asleep. The thought of being anywhere near him repulsed me. Not only that, but I started to feel terribly anxious as well as being scared. Scared for our son.

One evening David turned to me and questioned if I was scared of him. I responded in the positive, slowly nodding, wondering why he was asking.

He gently touched my face with his hand and said, 'That pleases me very much.'

Nasty mind games were his specialty.

2007

Angus was three months old when I was diagnosed with severe post-natal depression. I was vaguely keeping a mind's eye on it and sure enough the signs started exposing themselves.

Angus was developing plagiocephaly, a flat spot on the right side of his head, so when I gave him tummy time his neck muscles were not as strong as the maternity health nurse had hoped. I'd booked him in to see a paediatric osteopath and she said that if he didn't improve within the next few weeks of seeing her then he would have to be placed in a helmet to even out his skull. On the way home, I felt overcome with a wave of anger. I was envisaging David telling me that the whole thing was 'a load of crap', that she was just trying to make money from me. To him everyone was the enemy. The thought of not helping our son brought me to a rage. I was that lost in thought that it wasn't until I looked into my rear-view mirror I realised I'd run a stop sign being held by bloke in a road traffic block. It was lucky I didn't collide with an asphalt machine.

Once home, I was ready to start defending our child but, thankfully, David was still asleep. When he did emerge from the bedroom at 2 pm I had finally calmed down. Something was not correct with my thinking, though, as I'd reverted to considering leaving Angus with David, getting in my car and running into a tree to take my life.

I made an appointment to see my local doctor. When my time came to sit in his office, I told him of wanting to end my life. I told him of the animosity I was feeling for David. Bizarrely enough, I said there was really no reason for me to be angry because he was an extremely supportive husband. It was truly defensive and delusional all at once. How I could lie like that just to pretend that everything was perfect at home? Thank goodness, due to my medical history and my age, the doctor didn't take what I said I was planning to do lightly, neither with my car nor with myself in it. The CAT team from our local hospital was on our doorstep that afternoon, much to David's horror.

The Crisis Assessment Treatment team is a team of healthcare professionals that provide assessments during psychiatric crisis and short-term home treatment as an alternative to hospital. I'd told David they were coming over but when I invited the two psychiatric nurses in, he, without saying a word, headed out a side door, slamming it as he exited. He was in a complete rage. I knew I'd feel the full brunt of his anger when they left but I was so very grateful that the nurses were there to help me. I was at a dead end and didn't know who to turn to. Very quickly I was giving up hope.

During the few hours they were there, they spoke with me to assess what danger I felt I was to myself and/or to Angus. I clearly recall telling them of the anger I was feeling but instead of mentioning David I told them that I was scared I was turning into my mother. I was turning the anger on myself. When they asked who I thought my mother was I explained.

'She's a pathetic woman who does everything for my dad. She put up with so much bullshit from him and I hated her for not having the guts to look after my brother and me. It offended Dad that we invaded his life.'

I strongly felt how much I hated my parents, then the realisation hit me full on: I hated that I was married to a man who resembled my father. These narcissistic men who have to be in charge and be right, these sanctimonious sons of arseholes who bully women to gain nothing but to torment. I could see life from a different angle for the first time and it made me sick to think of how my mother never defended her children. Instead, she left us to try in vain to defend ourselves. How could she do that? I did have all the answers myself but continually questioned my thoughts because I never believed in myself. The more I spoke with them the more everything was falling into place within my mind. It made sense how I ended up with a man who treated me with such contempt and hatred. They wanted me to take new antidepressants and advised that Angus and I enter hospital for monitoring. As it was the public system, there was a waiting list.

After the nurses left, convinced that I was no harm to Angus or myself, David stormed back in the house, screaming and accusing me of bringing strangers into his home. I'd overridden his position as the man of the house and he was enraged. Angus was swaddled, asleep in my arms and I let David get it out of his system. His spite just flowed over me. I knew he would eventually get in his car and drive off, leaving us alone in peace, as was his pattern.

As the public health system was and always will be backed up, I was placed on a waiting list. I was on top of that list but I still had to wait my turn to be admitted and that's when Scarlett introduced me to a specialised psychologist in postnatal depression. Her name was Dr Lisa and when we met I didn't realise how much it would change my life on many levels.

I invited her into my home on a freezing winter's morning while David was asleep. I was so depressed I very rarely left the house unless it was work related, so she kindly came to me instead.

I knew that David would again lose his temper knowing that I was seeing someone without his say so.

Our first meeting was hard for me as I was worried about leaving the house and I was terribly scared David would wake up. The visit was shrouded in secrecy. I thought I'd be yelled at again. I was constantly scared. It was the simple act of her coming into my space, listening to my fears and understanding what I needed to get through a terrible time with a small baby. I just needed to feel assisted on the journey of being a new mother; it was that simple.

Within a couple of weeks, Angus and I were finally admitted to Banksia, a public psychiatric hospital in Heidelberg. It catered for mums going through major postnatal depression to get them the support they required. We spent a fortnight there. I saw counsellors, psychologists and psychiatrists on a daily basis, but I never mentioned David's behaviour or what I was going through at home. I loved being away from him though; it was like a holiday, only less luxurious.

The day I was hospitalised I was introduced to a very well known and admired professor of psychiatry. She was overseeing my medication and she had the sense of a peanut to tell me, while I was in a very fragile state of mind, because I had been on so many medications during my years with no success that she was at a loss. Placing her right index finger on her lips and a thumb to support her chin she spoke.

'Mmm, what am I going to do with you, Jackie? I really don't know what's going to help you out. I'm at a complete loss actually. Leave it with me.'

As I clenched my hands out of pure bewilderment, I looked at her with my calm mask on. My immediate thought was not so calm nor were the words swirling around my head. *Shit, you're an esteemed professor, I'm fucked if you can't work it out.*

At Banksia, the only contact with the outside world was an old phone in the reception area. After meeting with the professor, I needed to talk to someone, anyone – I was desperate. I called Mum. Big mistake.

Mum and Dad were in the afterglow of hosting a charity luncheon so they'd had a few drinks. As soon as she answered my call I knew I should have hung up.

'Hi, Mum. It's me, Jack.'

'Hi, sweetie. How's hospital? Oh, hang on, darling, sorry. I'm in the middle of hosting this luncheon and I'm a bit busy but here, speak with Mrs Taylor. I was only telling her and everyone at the table how wonderfully you've taken to motherhood.'

She knew damn well I wasn't coping with postnatal depression.

'No, Mum ... I need to speak with you ... Mum. *Mum!*'

I was then telephonically handed around the whole dining table to every woman who sat there. They'd all had way too many bottles of chardonnay.

I lost it. I felt I couldn't win. David didn't visit me and Mum wouldn't talk to me. I was surrounded within my immediate family by idiots. Worst of all, I shared the same DNA with a few of them. All of a sudden, security turned up telling me to hang up the call as I was distressing the other patients. Me! What about my family who had been distressing me for years? Where was the logic in that?

Angus and I were collected by David after fourteen days and returned home on another new medication that allowed me to sleep better but didn't alter my state of mind. I was still having manic moments and constant self-talk in my head, but Angus was my saving grace. I took to being a mother like I would never have imagined. It was a role that saved me. I became more aware and present of what I was doing rather than allowing my head to control the general narrative. I always thought of him first and what was best for him no matter the internal chatter.

In November, I worked up the courage to tell David I'd been seeing Dr Lisa. Out of the goodness of her heart she'd never charged me for her time, as she knew I couldn't afford it and David would never allow me to pay for it. I never did mention to him our meetings at the house. I told him that she wanted him to join in on my counselling sessions. He immediately became angry and defensive, swinging his hand near my face, willing to hit me, standing millimetres away. He accused me of going behind his back again.

All I wanted was help to feel better, to be able to cope and be a better mother to our son. After a few days he accepted, as I told him that she was very interested in his feelings and his opinion on how to help me. Remembering what she had told me, I instilled in him that I was the problem and I was in desperate need of his input. That caught his attention in a positive way. It made him feel in control again. When the day finally arrived, Dr Lisa explained some ground rules in the most subtle of ways.

She said that, by going through counselling together, there was a possibility that I could come to a point where there were two options in the conclusion of the counselling. Either I would want to, with support from him, save our marriage, or I could decide that I wanted to leave the marriage altogether. He agreed to attend the sessions for the following four months. He even had his own solo sessions with her.

When David joined the sessions he never hesitated in telling her that I was the problem of everything. He told her he adored me but that my family were terrible to me and tried to control everything I did. He said I was naive and he was trying to protect me from people who took advantage of me. It sickened me hearing this because it never made any sense. I never had his respect or support.

When it was my turn to talk, I felt this enormous pain in my throat, as if something were stuck in it. I couldn't speak properly, but it was a feeling of finally finding my voice. Unfortunately, because I was so hurt by past events in my life, the tears flowed to a point where I was hyperventilating, making it extremely difficult for anyone to understand me. David used it as an opportunity to explain to Dr Lisa that it was all in my mind.

'See? She's fucking losing it. She's completely mad.'

Thank goodness she understood my position.

Tears flowed for all the people who I had hurt and disappointed – my family and friends. I'd been so naive in my behaviour. I was disgusted in myself and my actions. I cried for my son and for the person that I felt he had inherited as a mother; I felt like a complete and absolute disaster as a human being. I didn't have an answer to why I felt like such a fucked up individual but in my heart I wanted to be the best mother he could have ever wished for.

There is a saying in the failed relationship arena that it takes two to tango and not for one moment did I feel I never had a role to play in the breakdown of the marriage. If anything, most of the time I took it all on as my fault as this was to be my second failed attempt at matrimony.

Dr Lisa revealed another side that she had uncovered. She let me know during a personal session that she felt David was hiding things from her during their talks and she was able to confirm his behaviour was not only in my head. His arrogance was showing through to her as if he wanted her to know he was in charge, willing her to push him. The more she listened to him the more he was painting a picture that wasn't pretty and logically didn't add up. Even though I had found a new sense of who I could be, I was still scared of leaving due to his unpredictable actions. I knew that time was no longer on my side but I was still hanging on. I knew David was unwilling to accept any role within what was, from my perspective, an absolute sham of a union. It was around this time I'd developed more clarity.

I'd killed off my friendship with Clair, all because of David. I missed her company terribly and just as I thought I had lost the chance of repairing my closest friendship, fate crossed my path. On a Sunday morning, on my way into the doctor's, two missionaries in crisp white shirts on pushbikes caught my eye. They were from my old church – the church I'd attended with Clair. It was a clear sign to make contact.

The following day, I drove over to her home unannounced and knocked on the front door with butterflies in my stomach and a bunch of flowers in my hand. When she opened the door, she stared for a moment not recognising me.

Before she could say anything, Angus, being the little socialite he was, walked past her, said, 'Yellow' (his toddler way of saying hello) and strolled inside like he owned the place. He headed off to play with Clair's boys. Really, she never had a choice in not allowing me in her home.

After a cup of tea and small talk, I humbly and wholeheartedly apologised to her for the pain I had caused. From that day on we have never been far away in distance or communication. I was welcomed back into her family with loving arms. I felt so very grateful indeed, as she's my sister.

Clair finally had the pleasure of meeting David just before we separated. After I told him that I had made contact with her all he could say in a threatening tone was, 'Be very careful, Jack. You don't know what you're getting yourself into. She's an alpha when it comes to relationships and she'll overpower you again.'

It was just another example of why I'd lost all respect for him. Our marriage was falling apart – we both knew it. When it would come to parting ways, it wasn't going to be as mutual as I hoped.

2008

I was living in a marriage that was not only decaying around me but I was also starting to feel my old hypomanic ways bubble up from inside. It was a horrific union and my repressed feelings were starting to leech out. The environment was making me sick and even if I wasn't thinking of myself anymore, I knew that it was not an appropriate home for Angus to be raised in. I decided to have all my hair cut off so it mirrored how I felt inside: ugly. I wanted to be invisible because whenever David looked at me, he'd just snigger, looking down at me in disgust. I started to drink again, when Angus was asleep and I was alone. It was my only support; it alleviated my fear.

It was quite poignant that on a beautiful evening in February, as the sun was going down, David and I were sitting in the family room after I'd put Angus to bed. One minute everything was calm, and then David noticed that I was reading a book and asked why I was wearing glasses. I froze, nervously answering his questioning. I didn't understand why he was asking in such a slowed tone. He got up from the couch and left the room, only to return with the Visa card statement. He walked over to where I was sitting and, imposing his 187 centimetre frame over mine, he started screaming at the top of his voice.

'WHERE THE FUCK DO YOU GET OFF BUYING A PAIR OF GLASSES ON MY CREDIT CARD?'

He'd given it to me two months prior in my name for Christmas gifts as my mother-in-law had berated him for not buying his son gifts in the past. I tried to stay calm and explain to him that I couldn't read without them. With each word of his reply, he hit me back and forth with an open palm across my head.

'You dumb fucking bitch! You can't read anyway!'

I snapped. I broke. It literally felt like a rubber band had been finally pulled to its maximum length. I couldn't take his abusive behaviour anymore; a major shift had occurred and I felt it within my mind. I yelled at the top of my voice.

'NO.'

I tried to get up from my seat. He pushed me back, digging his fingers into my shoulder to stop me leaving. I attempted to escape again and was successful. I ran into our ensuite, locking the door. I dropped to the ground, wrapped my arms tightly around my knees. A noise arose from my mouth that I had never made in all my life. It was that of a pained and wounded animal. It scared the hell out of me and I sat there on the cold floor, my face streaming with tears, almost convulsing. I couldn't stop shaking. I returned to the state of being a scared child, being yelled at by my father; it was truly surreal. I just kept repeating, 'No, no, no,' over and over. I was broken, I couldn't do it any longer, and with that it ended. Another marriage broken. I felt I had failed my son, but I was empty and exhausted. I had nothing left to give and I thought because I didn't have any money I couldn't leave; but I didn't care.

Over the years he'd taken away any wages I'd received, as well as my credit card. I had to come up with money for anything else Angus and I required. I begrudgingly handed him 240 dollars every week. I bought weekly groceries and he'd eat everything within a couple of days so we were left with nothing to eat. If we ever went out, he'd pay but when we got home, he pushed me to reimburse him and I did. I never received gifts from him for my birthday, Mother's Day or Christmas. He'd only buy things for our home, calling them 'tokens of his love'. Flywire screens, curtains, paint, carpet, stones to go in retaining walls and soil for the garden, even small hardware items from Bunnings were tallied up. I never received anything personal as a rule. David would take any money Angus received from relatives – every single cent and it was never seen again.

My mother-in-law Emmie was drip-feeding me cash to survive. We both knew if David found out I'd be punished for it. It was never spoken about, she just handed me cash when I visited alone with Angus.

I never knew that being exposed to living this way was deemed as financial abuse. Even when Angus was close to being born, I had to ask my mum to go shopping with me to buy baby clothes. David saw it as a waste and I was so scared to question him. A baby shower had never been on the cards, as David thought it was showing off. Visits from people became non-existent, as they knew they weren't welcome because of his behaviour. I was a married woman, living in a big home in a very affluent Melbourne suburb and I was penniless even though I worked full-time. Go figure! It's not as rare as people think.

And now I felt nothing. I was only grateful that for all that I had been through that night and with all the yelling and screaming Angus never woke up from his sleep. Or at least I told myself that. Subconsciously though I wasn't sure. He was just a toddler and no matter what his size or age, he'd been living amongst parents who were completely dysfunctional when together. No matter how much I tried to protect him and pretend everything was fine, kids pick up on what's going on.

Exhausted, the following day I drove Angus to his childcare centre and went straight home to start packing my car. I felt terribly embarrassed from my behaviour the previous night but I honestly reacted to what I was being put through for the umpteenth time. I knew I had until midday to pack as David slept most days until 1 pm. When he finally emerged from our bedroom, I was still packing and he was not as supportive of my leaving as I had previously thought. He started yelling at me for being a lazy bitch for not at least washing the dishes before I left his house.

'Fuck off to wherever you want but you're leaving my son to live with me. Go have a fucking breakdown somewhere else.'

I was exhausted. I let him rant and didn't try to defend myself. As he didn't get the attention he wanted, he then came into the room, yelling at me to get out of the house. He towered over me again, spitting with anger. I knew I was in trouble, so I tried then to push past him. Big mistake. He saw that as a challenge to push me back. As he was twice my weight with a body full of testosterone-charged rage, he grabbed my shoulders and slammed me backwards into a large framed print that was hanging on the wall behind me. My head went through the glass, hitting the wall, and shards rained over my head and shoulders.

Luckily, the glass only sliced one a patch of my hair off. I found my footing. Out of a fight or flight response, I only had the first option as he wouldn't let me go. In anger I tried to push past him again, but he overcame me and threw me on to the bed. I was screaming for him to get off as one of his knees held my legs and another reached up to my chest. He kept bouncing and shaking me, yelling at me to calm down. He looked completely possessed, and thinking of it now I probably looked very similar. I didn't want this arsehole overpowering me again – this time I was leaving. I was under his full body weight with both of his hands on my throat and I thought he was going to either strangle me or break my ribs.

I remembered something that my midwife Alice said to me during the birth of Angus. It's truly insane that in a split second an idea of weight ratio can return to you. She told me that instead of yelling – a reaction to the pain of labour – to channel my energy into pushing. So I did just that. I stopped yelling and instead used my energy in more positive way. I used the leverage of him bouncing me on the bed and the adrenalin I was feeling to pull one of my knees free and up to his groin. It hit him with such force in the balls that he released me. It was long enough for me to scramble into the kitchen, grab our home phone and dial 000.

As the operator asked me who I wanted to be connected to, David came hobbling up after me, his face contorted.

'Ambulance, fire brigade or police?' She waited for my response. I gave her none.

There was a vision in my head of Granny Emmie, David's mother, telling me not to make a scene, as it would be an embarrassment to the whole family.

David stared desperately, whispering, telling me to put the phone down. 'Jack, put it down, please, put it down.'

I disconnected the call, dropping the phone to the ground. Tears were rolling down my face. I was lost and empty. I made my way to the front door feeling completely deflated. I told David that I'd be returning for the remainder of my things once he left for work. It was then I understood why I had been advised to plan leaving the marital home. It wasn't merely to tick a box; it was an essential point of a safe exit.

He felt threatened and provoked by my leaving and he was in no way going to allow me to go quietly – his ego wouldn't allow it. As I drove away, I could feel the adrenalin flowing through me and one part wished he had have hit me, bruising me so badly that the pain I was feeling inside could be seen by all on the outside. I had to pull over to the roadside and cry. I had to let myself feel what I'd just experienced. Psychological scarring can hurt so much more than the physical scars that can heal over days and weeks, eventually invisible as the body restores and heals itself.

2009

Once I'd collected my thoughts and calmed down enough to get back on the road, I collected Angus from his childcare centre and dropped him off at my parents. I then headed straight to my solicitor's office – a 60 kilometre round trip in a dazed state.

I'd been thinking of leaving David for a while so I sought a solicitor a few months prior just to cover my bases. My first thought back then was that I could go through Legal Aid, as I didn't have any money to pay for legal advice. That was very wrong of me to assume. Once I was interviewed by one of their lawyers, they told me because my name was on our family's house title and the property was valued at over 400,000 dollars – Legal Aid's cap – I wasn't eligible to be represented by them. Instead, they gave me a list of family law solicitors to contact who may be able to represent me. That is how I met and engaged Margo to be my legal representative; a solicitor and a barrister who would guide me through the Victorian Family Court if it ever came to that – and it would.

I understand that a lot of people who engage legal representation throughout their separation process are not necessarily happy with who they have representing them, but I must have hit the jackpot.

Representing myself was never on the table – that takes too much emotional management. Cutting corners wasn't an option either – finding a solicitor who specialised in a different area (for example, conveyancing) might have saved me money, but it wouldn't have been worth it. As I was in Victoria, my first half an hour interview with the solicitor was free. This was almost like a speed date – I got a sense of whether they had my best interests in mind, in and out of court. I personally found Margo to be a very level headed woman with a good dry sense of humour, which I liked. When I got over-emotional, she was there to calm me down and help me breathe through it. She'd explain to me the hoops that I would have to jump through at times to keep the Family Court happy. It was all about one step at a time.

No matter what I'd been through, David wouldn't be put on trial, as the Family Court only then operated on what is best for the children. He wasn't going to be put on trial for his behaviour towards me and that was at times enormously frustrating. When things did start getting overwhelming for me, my sister Jane accompanied me for support.

I had to return to my parents as I felt I had nowhere else to go. Living with them while they yelled at each other after drinking each night was excruciating. The night Dad started banging on my door and yelling at me was one of the scariest.

'Get your fucking act together or get out!'

I was holding onto Angus so closely in bed, trying to cover his little ears so he couldn't hear. Thinking I had no other choice, I panicked. The next day I packed my car again and headed back to David.

I like to think of it as the Pinball Move. Think of yourself as the tiny silver ball sitting in the pinball machine – game on! Imagine the way that ball is pushed and shoved and shunted into other spaces but, before it can rest after a downward run, it's knocked into another status of unrest again, and then it repeats.

On average, a woman will leave and/or return to an abusive relationship seven times before she leaves for good, if at all. I never knew this and returned with my son in my arms, defeated. Margo called me, gently trying to guide me back on the path of logic but I just couldn't deal with it; it felt so alien to me. It was all too much for me to deal with and I left my job – another fail. My boss knew what was going on but I cut her off too. I discarded anyone who could connect me to failure, anyone who could view me as anything but normal.

David let me in the house after I practically begged him and I headed straight to the kitchen to make another meal that would probably end up being put in the rubbish bin again. At least I knew what was ahead of me. He followed me, screaming into my face while I held on to Angus, covering his head to protect him.

'Why the fuck are you back? Have you had your fucking breakdown? Leave my boy with me. He's mine.'

I breathed through it as I'd done in the past, stayed calm and hoped he'd stop after a while. I could survive his abuse. I'd done it up to this point so what was different? Outside the front door was unpredictable; my abuser wasn't.

It wasn't long before my mania began to rise up again. The urgency to leave had begun outweighing the need to stay. I was in fight or flight, seesawing back and forth, spinning round and round.

Stay? Don't stay? I can't afford to leave. How do I get money to leave? If I don't stay where do I go?

Everything was accentuated. Sleeping was difficult. My new place to lie at night was on an old musty mattress in Angus' room. It gave me peace knowing I was next to him, keeping him safe. I was low to the ground and felt small, and that's what I wanted. Small and irrelevant is how I felt. Staring up at the colourful fluorescent stars stuck on my baby's roof, a magnificent idea sprung to mind. It was brilliant – my answer to earning money. I don't know why I hadn't thought of it earlier. I presumed good coin too. Considering my options whilst listening to my child softly breathe, I eventually closed my eyes.

The next morning, after feeding Angus and getting him off to day care, I started thumbing through the Yellow Pages and circling escort services. Here was my logic: I was going to start doing something that I hoped I'd enjoy, something I missed terribly. I missed being touched, being loved. But people would have to pay for it. I couldn't bring myself to meet random people at a club. I was a person who would visit a library for fun. Reading was fun; picking up men in a bar was not. I could say I was too prudish to go hunting for sex but that would in itself be the definition of an oxymoron. I presumed I could bring in a valuable sum to support the two of us, better than I'd ever brought in before. And my favourite reason: I was going behind David's back BIG time. I was going to do something that in his wildest mind he would never consider me doing.

After nervously chatting with a lovely lady on the phone for five minutes I had booked in a time to meet with her the following day. I excitedly started organising what I was going to wear. I picked out a black business suit and heels. As Friday morning arrived, I took Angus to Granny Emmie's home. I waved goodbye from the patio. I told Emmie I was going for a new job interview. I didn't tell her what type of interview it was though.

It gave me such a thrill knowing that I was doing something so electrifying. The build-up was intense and I was high. I drove to a car park in Flinders Street and excitedly walked to my appointment on busy Swanston Street, Melbourne. Everyone I walked by had no idea what was going on in my crazy mind. It was like I had a secret mission.

Once I'd arrived I took a jolted trip in a dilapidated lift two floors up. I entered a foyer that was very tired, looking for apartment 202. I took a deep breath and pushed the grubby doorbell. The sturdy solid door was unlocked and then opened by a blonde lady in her fifties. Her name was Cat. I introduced myself and she let me in to the smoke-hazed hall. I followed her on the worn lino; so old it was back in fashion, retro from the 1940s. The front of the room looked down on to the bustling street below. The windows were old – deteriorated thin glass framed by old sills with peeling paint. All I could hear were trams and buskers. I was introduced to the receptionist, a young girl named Libby.

I looked around at the deteriorating brown vinyl couches and threadbare ottoman in the adjoining room. Tea and coffee were in labelled plastic containers on top of a bar fridge. We sat at the old table they worked on, files and bills scattered. It had to be from the 1920s. It was art deco – its varnish had dulled. Cat started by explaining that she did the books for the business, then offered me coffee.

'Ah, no thanks. I'd probably spill it over myself. I'm a tad nervous. So no, but thank you.'

I felt like an eager child who didn't want to make a mistake.

She then asked me what brought me to her establishment. It wasn't a weird question but one I had to think about. I'd rehearsed something but I just blurted out the truth.

'I'm a single mum living under my ex-husband's roof. I just need enough money to leave.'

She raised her thinly pencilled eyebrows and nodded. I could see it didn't surprise her. 'We have a hell of a lot of women on the books and if they were to walk through here now, you'd probably know a few of their faces. We have actors, nurses, uni students – the lot. Don't worry, you're not alone. It's a common story. One of my girls, Brittany, is about to come off night shift. She's a computer engineer. Doesn't need the money, she just enjoys it. Please don't be embarrassed.' She continued. 'OK, let me explain what happens and you can get a feeling if escorting is something you'd like to do.'

She began by handing me a black binder. Inside was obviously something that maybe Libby had put together on a quiet day. It was a paper version of a PowerPoint presentation. Elite Ladies was set up to reflect a classier side to escorting. All girls who were contracted to them had to wear unscuffed high heels and stockings were mandatory – they were to be worn with a suspender belt at all times. No chipped nail polish either. Everything had to look highly presentable.

She commented that the outfit I'd worn was perfect. Oddly enough, I felt proud I'd passed the first requirement. My dress had to be business-like so as not to stand out if I were to enter one of Melbourne's better hotels. You didn't want to be stopped by security or a concierge unless they'd arranged you for one of their guests. Anything lacy and satin was an obvious requirement for underwear. It was my choice of colour unless I was to visit a client who was of Indian descent; word was they loved red, orange and hot pink. Definitely no black – that was for mourning only.

I was to organise a small toiletry bag that would fit into my handbag. Everything had to be a mini version. I was to carry a handbag not a suitcase. Priceline was about to make a small fortune from me. My bag would include the following:

- Listerine and mints for fresh breath, especially for smokers. I wasn't one and thank goodness I wasn't expected to kiss a client's mouth, because fucking them was so much better! (Don't worry the irony played out in my manic mind immediately.)

- A small hairbrush.

- Dry shampoo for an easy quick fix.

- A scrunchie to keep my hair dry in the shower in case a hotel shower cap wasn't available.

- Body wash. I would shower before I slept with a client and straight after each visit before leaving a client's room.

- Hand towel.

- A mini bag of my makeup essentials including cotton pads and tips. No makeup smears allowed.

- Two spare pairs of thigh stockings for emergency. No holes allowed. ('You never know if a client will get rough and accidently rip them.')

- Perfume – nothing cheap.

- Baby wipes.

The salacious part of the tool kit wasn't urgent, except the first request:

- Condoms. The thinner the better. Flavoured, as it could make the process of putting them on a client more palatable.

- A sponge for when I got my period. This request left me lost for words. It didn't compute – I envisioned a CHUX Superwipe, which wasn't right. It was a sea sponge, but clean. Reason: if I got my period, I was to insert it into my vagina so I could continue to work. I couldn't logistically work out how it would be removed!

- Different sizes of butt plugs – a gadget I never knew existed, and had to have explained to me. Who'd have known? Now I do and wish I didn't!

- Basically any sex toy that existed that's sole purpose was to bring pleasure, or pain, depending on the clients wants and needs.

I would be expected to work at least one night on the weekend, as that's when Melbourne comes to life with travellers from interstate. I'd be given a driver/bodyguard for the first three weeks, unless it was a city job that I could catch public transport to. After that I could take bookings from home and make my own way there. I needed an ABN and my hourly rate was to be 350 dollars, minus a third for the house and public transport costs. As a contractor I could get a tax deduction on all goods related to the job. That one got me thinking about how the hell I was going to explain it to my family accountant. Thinking quickly, I thought it best head down to the local H&R Block kiosk at my shopping centre in the future.

Cat asked me to stay and hang around as long as I wanted to meet some of the other girls and ask any other questions I had. I met three girls before I left. Sally was a lyricist whose philosophical views on the current state of music royalties were astounding. She was also studying teaching at Monash University. Kayden was a nurse at The Royal Children's Hospital and a single mother with two small boys. I was dumbfounded she'd have any energy left for sex. Then there was Lexi. She was from Ballarat and she also worked as a dancer at The Gentlemen Gallery in Lonsdale Street. She told me that even though she made better money escorting, she enjoyed the camaraderie of the club environment more. She did most of her sex work bookings from home and it got a bit lonely at times. Her father was a high-ranked police officer in her hometown so she moved to Melbourne to escape his repressive ways. Everyone knew who she was in that part of country Victoria and she just wanted to disappear. I asked the girls what their biggest worry was about being in the industry and they all pretty much agreed it was seeing girls putting the majority of their earnings up their noses, trying to muffle their grief from past bad experiences. It could be a soul-destroying job if you weren't careful.

Just before I left, Cat let me know that she could definitely offer me work as soon as I was ready. I wanted to start on Monday but there were a few things I had to do before I could begin my new career. I had to choose a name – no one was to ever use their own name once working, not even when answering a call from Cat. I was trying to think of something exotic when a small voice came from the corner. It was Libby.

'It should be Grace. She looks like a Grace.'

And so, Grace it was – not at all avant-garde but everyone agreed.

'Thank you, Libby, that's very kind of you to say,' I replied. And I meant it. In recent times, I felt like the sea witch Ursula from *The Little Mermaid*.

Just before I could finish polite conversation, I was whipped back to reality by Cat again.

'You'll also need to bring in a certificate from your doctor to clear you of any STDs.' She continued. 'If you don't want to go to your family doctor for obvious reasons, I can organise an appointment with a female doctor in Collingwood we've been using. She's safe. Unfortunately, some of the girls have had bad experiences with male doctors in the past. A few have made them feel really vulnerable, either through guilt or by inappropriately touching them. People think because you're a sex worker you're up for anything in your spare time. It's not good.'

I was absolutely buzzing and wanting to please my new friends. I've been told when I'm manic or on a downward spiral my family and friends can read it in my eyes. Dilated irises mean I'm on a naturally produced chemical high. If I'm spiralling down, the whites of my eyes appear yellow. If Cat had noticed me that day she must have thought I'd been doing drugs. My senses were so incredibly heightened.

Leaving my new place of work that afternoon, I stepped back out onto the street and caught a tram down Collins Street to Jane's work at NAB's head office in windy Docklands. I went to front reception asking if she could be called downstairs. I was bursting with excitement that I couldn't hold inside any longer. Minutes later she stepped out of a lift into the beautifully designed foyer. We took a seat on an oversized plush lounge near a south-facing window.

'Wow. Hi. What a surprise. What are you doing here? Oh my God, are you OK? Where's Angus?'

'Bloody hell, Jane, calm down! You're worse than me at the moment. Everything's fine. I have something exciting to tell you. Well, I think it's exciting. I don't know if you will.' I sensed that she mightn't see my vision. I started. 'I have a new job.'

'That's fantastic. What is it?' she replied, with a broad smile on her face.

Pursing my lips, I answered. 'You're going to have to guess. Go on, I'll give you three.' I was brimming with joy.

'Retail?'

'No. Guess again.'

'Merchandising? Please let it be that. You're so talented.'

I saw that she wasn't going to guess. I mean, why would she? I was on planet Saturn and she was sitting in Docklands.

She was so straight-faced, her tone almost a whisper. 'Jack, what's going on? You seem almost high. Where are you working? Tell me.'

'In the city. Not far from here. We can have lunch together!' My speech was picking up speed again. I felt she was close to guessing. It scared but enthralled me at the same time. My pulse was thumping harder. 'I'm OK. I have a job and I'm starting Monday.'

I wasn't starting Monday but it was as though I was willing it. I was like a child who was about to have something truly special ripped away from me.

'I've met new friends and I know I'll be happy.'

'Jackie what is it? What's the job? Tell me now.'

'I've got a job with an escort agency.'

'Sorry?' Tilting her head forward, Jane's eyes widened as though she hadn't heard me correctly.

'I've decided to become a sex worker. The money is good and I can leave David and raise Angus on my own. I can move away from him, go interstate. We can start again, alone.'

Jane just stared at me. Her breathing picked up, but only enough for me to hear. It was as though she couldn't catch her breath. 'No.' She moved her head from side to side. 'No. Jack, no. You can't do this to Angus.'

I was amazed. 'Do it to him? I'm not doing anything to him. I'm helping us. I'll earn good money.'

'Not that way, Jack. You can't.' She kept her voice very low.

'Stop. Just stop. This is what I'm going to do. I will do it. You always say I can't do things. You think you're better than me and you're not.'

'Please don't do this, Jack. No.' She looked horrified.

'I'm going. Don't ruin it and don't tell Andrew. I told you but you have to keep it secret. No one is going to understand. It's OK. I'm going to be fine. I have to pick Angus up.'

Leaving her dazed in the foyer, I escaped through the thick-glazed revolving doors into the windy but sunny afternoon. I decided to walk to the car park, as a way to expel some of the adrenaline I was feeling. I had no idea how I was going to pay for new lingerie, sex toys and toiletries. I barely had enough money to pay Secure Parking to retrieve my car, but I'd think about that later.

Driving back to collect Angus, I stopped next to a car in congested traffic. A guy in the neighbouring vehicle briefly caught my eye and my thought was, *I'm an escort. I'm a sex worker and you have no idea. You're looking at me and all you see is a boring housewife but I'm a prostitute.* It was enormously thrilling.

It didn't take long after that for the first surge of guilt to hit me. I was high and felt it just as I turned onto the freeway, realising that Angus was going to have a prostitute for a mum. How could I tell him? He'd only just turned three. What would his little friends think? The thought stayed with me until I pulled into Emmie's driveway, but I was also so very excited to tell her the interview had gone well. I gave her some made-up business name and told her I was to start Monday.

As soon as I returned home, I started packing a few of Angus' things and got back in the car to drive to Mum's. I could feel the clouds rolling in. I was getting tired again – it was exhaustion setting in from the high I'd been on. David wouldn't miss us. I couldn't stand the thought of him degrading me again for not being able to get out of bed if it came to that, and it would.

The following day I was back in bed at Mum's house. She was only to come into my room Sunday morning to tell me I hadn't been answering my phone and Jane needed to speak with me straight away.

'I don't know what you've done but she sounded stressed and said it was important.'

As I dialled, I could smell smoke – it was so intense. I opened my curtain saw that a haze had settled.

Jane picked up my call. 'Jack, get dressed. You're to meet Andrew at Bailey's Café in Main Street at 10.30 this morning.'

'My throat hurts. Are you coming?' I was so tired.

'No. Everyone's throat is hurting at the moment. Stop being so dramatic and think of all the lives that have been lost while you've been sleeping. Don't be late.' She hung up.

Why was she so pissed off? Lives lost?

I got dressed and told Mum I'd be back to collect Angus, then got in my car and drove straight to the café. I was waiting at a small table when my brother-in-law walked in with a straight face. I greeted him first.

'Why is it so smoky? The haze is hurting my eyes.' I kept drinking water.

'You haven't heard, have you?' Unimpressed, he continued. 'Jane said you've been asleep since Friday night. There were terrible fires through the state yesterday. They are still counting the deaths. King Lake, Marysville and more. Burnt to nothing.'

I was stunned. I'd just spent a weekend in Marysville with Clair for my fortieth. A beautiful little town, now gone.

Our drinks arrived. Andrew took his spoon and started stirring, then he began. 'Jack, Jane told me about your decision to start a new job tomorrow, a "new career".'

The dry sarcasm in his voice hurt. I didn't say anything.

He continued. 'I invited you here to let you know how upset we are. I want you to know how much your behaviour has hurt her. She can't deal with you anymore, your erratic, senseless conduct.' There was an emphasis on the last words. 'If you decide to go into the city tomorrow and continue down this insane path, I am going to call Child Protection and have Angus removed. It's that simple.' Under his breath he calmly repeated his words more simply so I understood. 'Continue and you will lose your child. I will have him taken away. You have a choice. What are you going to do?'

By this stage there were tears rolling down my face. I hung my head in shame for what I'd done. I'd never felt so ashamed in my life. It was impossible to think I had put myself in a situation where my little boy could be removed from me.

'Do you have any idea how much danger you would be putting Angus in, let alone yourself? What were you thinking? What is wrong with you?

I remember feeling as though I couldn't breathe. There was a heaviness in my chest. I sat with this huge guilt that anyone would think I would do anything threatening to Angus. I would never do that to my child. Andrew could see my distress.

'Jack, your behaviour is getting worse. You need help. We're begging – you need to go back and see a psychiatrist. We love you; you're everything to Angus. You need to get better. Jane and I will help you.' He looked desperate for me to understand and put his hand on mine.

He followed me home back to Mum's, explaining that I needed to get some medical help immediately. I returned to bed to sleep until the following day when I received another visit from the CAT team. I was given medication to settle my awful state of mind. I was to start visiting my psychiatrist again the same week.

Andrew never spoke a word to anyone else about the chat Jane and I had the previous Friday or about his talk with me.

Two weeks later I met Jane and Andrew at Margo's office. I signed my medical power of attorney to Anne and my financial control to Jane. I understood I wasn't well enough to make any decisions and they wanted to help. The following week when I was feeling better, I returned with Andrew to my home while David was at work and finally packed Angus' and my things. We left nothing of ours behind apart from a few of Angus' clothes for when he had to visit his dad. I took nothing of David's. I didn't want any of it. I've always been able to hold a piece of clothing or effects and remember where and why I got it. The memories flood back. I wanted nothing to do with any of it.

I decided to call Margo the next day asking her to begin proceedings, telling her that I didn't want the house in settlement. David used to scream at me that he'd never part with 'his' house. I wanted nothing but what was I legally entitled to. I just needed enough to raise my little boy.

I felt well enough to visit Eastern Domestic Violence Outreach Service (EDVOS) as Margo called ahead explaining my situation and asked them to interview me in the hope of gaining emergency accommodation. Dad was back to his old ways again and I couldn't cope with raising Angus and dealing with his verbal abuse.

Still to this day, though, I never felt ashamed that I met the ladies at the escort agency. They were all extremely kind and patient with me because I really had no idea how I came across that day when I met everyone. To move forward I just put it down to experience. Feelings of guilt ran over me occasionally because of my behaviour but I had to learn to place them to one side and move ahead in a different direction. I was under no illusion that had David ever found out about what had occurred he would use it against me in court.

I fully support sex workers in our community. They work extremely hard to put, as we all do, food on the table and to live life. To be slut shamed or treated like second-class citizens is beyond my understanding.

Cat called me after my initial visit to the agency, asking if I'd reconsider starting. I politely declined. I told her that I'd decided escorting wasn't something I could see myself doing. She wished me all the best.

Another chapter closed. I'd had an experience at a place that my great-grandmother would have described as a bad house, full of bad women. I think not.

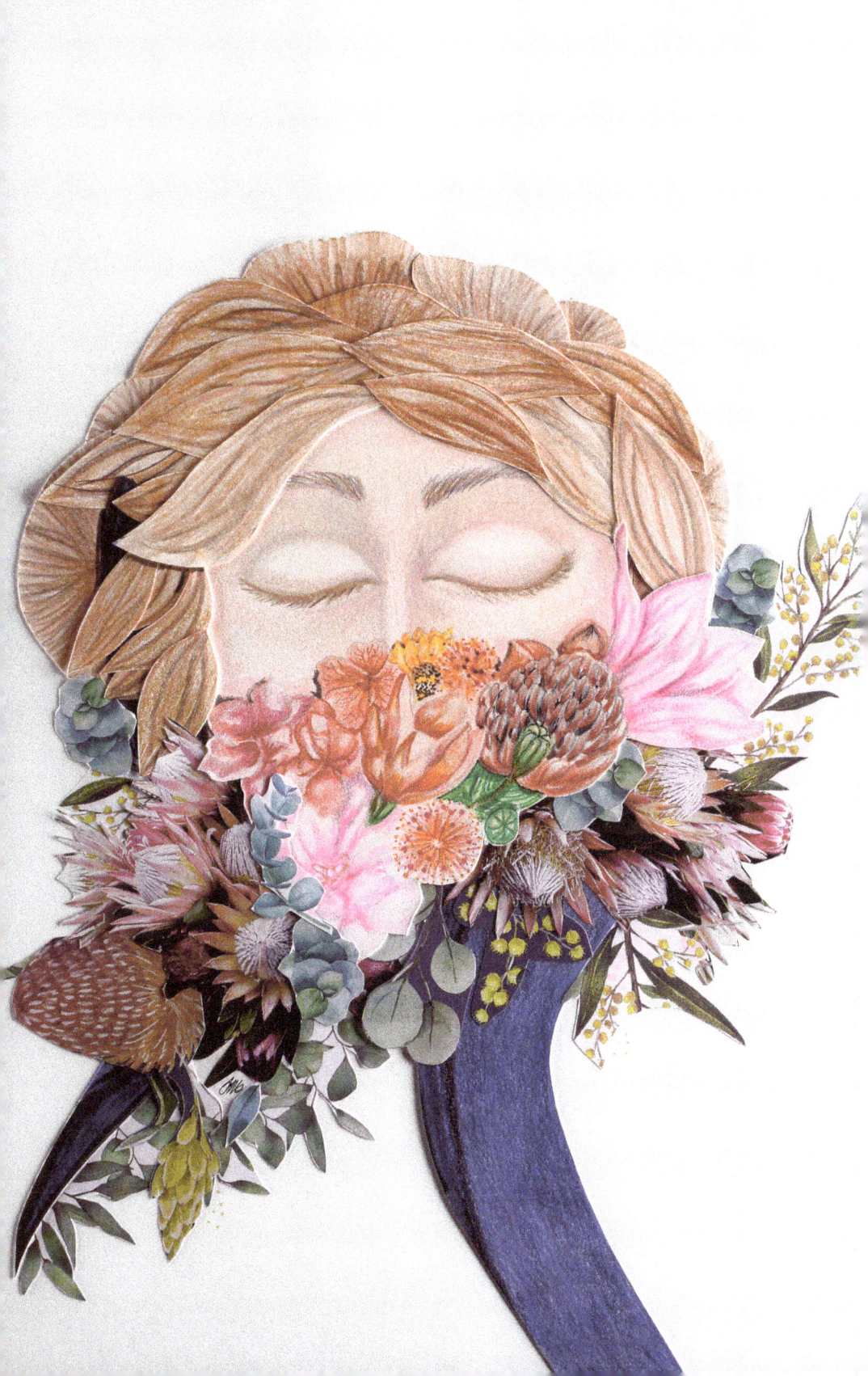

2010

My next lesson was to accept the path I needed to go down and try and end the cycle of abuse. Margo was my adviser regarding all things legal. She was realistic and logical; two things I lacked.

In private, David had written out an offer to give me 85,000 dollars over four years, paid in six payments per year. There was a caveat that if his business didn't turn over expected earnings it would be extended indefinitely. Margo said it was pure control and incredibly patronising. Before I met her, I didn't know what the legal system said I was due. When our meeting ended, she sent me immediately down to EDVOS.

'What number is it?' I asked.

'You don't need a number. Just walk down Broad Street and you'll see a blue building on your left. There won't be a sign, so just walk into the building and you'll see reception. They're expecting you.'

'Why hasn't it got a number?'

'Because it's a refuge for women and children escaping domestic violence. They don't want anyone knowing where they are.'

EDVOS is one of a few centres across Melbourne that supports women and children who are escaping domestic violence. I didn't initially understand why I was being sent to speak with a counsellor. Abuse had been such a big part of my life that I categorised it in my mind as normal behaviour. But it obviously wasn't. David had abused me, and my father before that. I'd endured years of emotional, financial and physical abuse.

Immediately on arriving I spoke with a lady who sat behind a bulletproof screen. She then let me through the heavy, locked security door. I was introduced to Robin. She was to be my new case manager who'd support me every step the way until the court proceedings were over. I returned to my parent's home for only a few days until EDVOS found us emergency accommodation.

Angus was so young but he already sensed something wasn't right and he kept asking for his dad. It didn't help that I was so on edge. David continually called me, asking where I was and when I was returning his son. He screamed down the line that I'd never get a cent. I was to get Angus back to him then I could, 'Fuck off.' When he'd verbally attack me, I still held the phone up to my ear and took it. To hang up on him wasn't an option – it would have been impolite. That's how out of kilter I was.

EDVOS receive multiple housing requests daily for accommodation from abused women and their children. As I was leaving to go back to Mum's to retrieve our belongings, my case manager asked me if I had any money to get by. I realised I didn't. Neither my bank account nor purse had any money in it as I'd spent everything I had over the past few weeks. I had no money for petrol or even enough to buy a packet of nappies for my son. I really felt like I hit rock bottom again that day.

Even though I was no longer living with David, I still felt the remnants of his control over me. I was scared to buy essentials, like petrol, in case I got in trouble. His mind games were still affecting me. Looking back now, I could see how things from the past still held power over me. One afternoon before we broke up, when we had six tradesmen working at our house. David was out, so I was home alone with them. They were chatting and enjoying a beer at the end of a hard day's work. I needed to go out and collect something for dinner, Angus was in my arms. As soon as I walked out the door and the men turned to me, I froze.

'I have to go down the street. Can I please go down the street?'

They all turned to face one another as though the bloke standing next to them was giving the answer.

'Um, sorry. Are you asking me?' One of the confused guys answered.

'I'm sorry yes, I'm asking if I can go down the street. I promise I won't be long.'

'Ahhh, love, you don't have to ask us if you want to go down the street. This is your home.'

I was at a loss as to why I needed to ask complete strangers to leave my own home but I did.

'Can I please go down the street?' I closed my eyes just willing them to say yes.

'Um, yeah I suppose so.' They looked so confused.

I didn't mean to embarrass anyone – I was just so used to David telling me what to do.

Moments like this still played out, even when I wasn't around David.

I didn't have a plan for my exit from my parents' home. I was too proud to ask anyone in my family for money; I had to fix it by myself. Robin gave me fifty dollars out of their petty cash tin and helped me call Centrelink. I secured an emergency appointment with a specialised department who helped women in need of financial help.

The final night before we entered the accommodation I couldn't sleep. At 2 am I got up and went into the lounge room. It was the same room where I'd offered David port the first time he'd come into my parents' home, the first time we'd slept together. The anger and grief I felt was so extreme. I couldn't see how our life was going to play out for Angus but I knew I was responsible for making it the best I could for the both of us. Society tells you that as a single mother you don't hold any value, especially if you don't work, but in real life we become tougher and stronger as individuals. There is no one else to lean on that can provide for your child as you can. I was it.

It wasn't easy to let go of the 'picket fence dream' I once had, or thought I had. Margo put a caveat on our home so David could not legally do anything to it, like sell it or damage it to lower its value, however, he did change all the locks on the doors. Eventually real estate valuers were brought in so they could settle on a figure for the house.

Thinking about the way David used to treat me and how I behaved around him sickened me. I couldn't cope with the idea of being anywhere near him now and he knew it. I was scared.

It wasn't long after Angus and I moved into our first accommodation that I had to notify my case manager that we had to move again. I didn't want David knowing where we were and one afternoon while I was in my car he drove past me in the opposite direction. I realised that we weren't very far from his place of business. I became so overwhelmed and I felt sure he'd seen me. I was worried he'd follow me home. Our location had to be kept a secret from my close friends and family, just in case word got out accidentally. If David had ever followed me to our safe house, I'd have been in a lot of trouble, not only personally, but because all of the other women would've been clearly upset by it.

I had Angus with me full-time. David didn't ask for custody of his child because something significant had been brought to light. On a few occasions when Angus was returned from David's care, we knew that he wasn't being looked after properly. His childcare teachers noticed that Angus was sometimes still wearing the same nappy I had dropped him off in at 9 am. I would take Angus to his childcare centre. David would then collect him at 10 am, take him home, then return him to childcare for me to collect him around 3.30 pm each weekday. Now, you can imagine what happens to a child's nappy after it's been worn for six hours or more and it never gets changed. Sometimes I would have to bath Angus immediately to remove dried up faeces. He would be red raw. It was beyond unacceptable. That kind of person doesn't deserve to look after a child. The Victorian Family Court saw differently though, even with evidence from childcare witnesses.

When we were still living with David, Angus started telling his teacher after he witnessed a boy hitting one of the girls in the centre, 'Daddy does that to my Mummy. Daddy hit Mummy.' I was called immediately to the director's office and questioned on whether or not David ever hit me. Astounded that anyone could know what was going on in our home, I answered in the negative, scared they would call Social Services and take Angus off me. When we eventually had our time in court, the childcare workers' evidence was used against me, as I'd told her David never hit me. I never blamed her; I was the one who lied. I did anything and everything to protect my family no matter what. I couldn't imagine what David would have done if I'd said yes as it would've been reported to the police as well.

We were relocated to our second emergency accommodation through the Salvation Army, closer to the city. The unit was very old and rundown but we made it our little home. Some nights we would go for a walk to the corner supermarket, Angus riding on an old little scooter Emmie had given him. I'd buy groceries for the night then make him dinner while he sat on the raggedy carpet watching Ben 10 and playing with matchbox cars from Mum. There were quite a few nights I'd be in the kitchen with tears streaming down my face because I was completely lost as to how this mess I'd gotten us into was going to end. I had no idea. It dawned on me to focus on the end result rather than being overwhelmed by fear itself, and it was an old-fashioned idea at that. I placed a large calendar on the kitchen wall so each night I could put a thick red line through the day. This helped me know that I was closer to it all being over and getting our life on track – hopefully a much brighter one.

With all the grief that we were going through there was a glimmer of something I hadn't anticipated. Being a single mother, Centrelink advised me that I could either stay at home or study. I felt so humbled that I had an opportunity to return to university. I went down and enrolled in Liberal Arts – the first step in getting into a course I now felt worthy of studying. I was able to enrol Angus into the on-campus childcare centre so I could check on him a couple of times during the day. I hoped that my course was a pathway entry into a BA in psychology. It was so empowering – I was given a second chance in education. I finished my year with distinctions and honours in selected units. I was proving to myself that I wasn't any of the names I'd been branded with in the past, not only by David but also by my parents. I wasn't stupid or hopeless. I could now be in an environment that allowed me to be inquisitive and expressive; one that built my confidence and didn't stifle it.

My brain was stretched to a point of exhaustion some days but I grew and developed so much as a person. I met some amazing people, one being a wonderful lecturer John Moutou. He taught me that I could do anything as long as my heart was in it. His wise words were written inside my lecture pad. *Education has the potential to free us from all enslaving dependences and addictions and can become the door to more self-relying living.* And that's what I wanted: to be self-reliant. A goal I strived for each day.

After one and a half years of legal toing and froing, we had our day in court. Before our time in front of the Family Court-appointed judge, I had the opportunity to witness the strangest thing I'd ever seen within the legal fraternity.

Margo appointed me a barrister and he asked to meet me in a large café two hours prior to proceedings. A very well dressed and well-spoken gentleman called James let me know calmly that David was sitting in the café too, away from view. I didn't understand what he was saying.

'Now, don't get upset, but David's with his barrister and is sitting at his table. Coffee?'

'What? No. What's happening?' I looked at Robin, my support case manager from EDVOS. I was completely confused – we were meant to meet in front of a judge.

'Jackie, if you're not comfortable, we can go.'

'Just tell me what's happening.' I was confused.

James finally filled me in. 'Before we meet in front of Judge Simmons today, David's barrister and I are going to have a bit of a chat and see if David will offer you a settlement.'

I was astonished. 'You are kidding me! Do you understand who I'm up against? He will never settle this early.'

He continued. 'Just trust me, Jackie. I'm going to try.'

Now, I have no idea how long it takes to become a barrister and I have no doubt that they are in general very intelligent people, but are they logical? I was thinking not. Thank goodness I didn't order coffee, I was hyper enough as it was. That was one and a half hours I'll never get back.

James went to David's table to speak with his barrister. He then returned with a counter offer. Every single offer was refuted by both parties. David was offering the most ridiculous amount to support our son. Then I started to open my eyes to what was going on around me. Swirling around our little table were barristers and legal representatives moving like excited ants, out and around different tables, back and forth. Each analytical mind was trying to act in their client's best interests before they were to stand in front of the judge.

We did end up meeting Judge Simmons, and we stood as our case number was read along with our names. Words were exchanged about what had been discussed in the café. It took no longer than ten minutes. All David's barrister, and he seemed a very intelligent and calm man, could say in his defence was that I was unfit to be a mother to our son because I had 'mental health issues' and had been married before. They claimed it was my ploy all along to take David's hard-earned money. I was officially branded a 'gold digger'. What they'd forgotten to mention was I'd walked away from my first marriage with nothing and I was prepared to do it a second time too, had it not been for my son. David knew this because it had been a reason two years prior to pull over our car on the Eastern Freeway and scream at me for not taking anything from Charlie.

His voice had screeched into my ear that I was leeching off him, adding I was fucking ugly and fat. That was his new poisonous rant tactic; my facial features and weight.

David's story also included that our relationship broke down two years prior to it actually ending. He told my solicitor we had nothing to do with one another so the monetary figure would be less. Judge Simpson was then presented with James' evidence of travel receipts, proving that David took Angus and I on a trip to Tasmania eighteen months prior. They went back and forth, until we were told to go away with counsel and work it out for the sake of Angus.

As we were leaving the courtroom, David's solicitor held the door open for me and, in the kindest tone, wished me luck. David sacked him that afternoon.

Once outside, he stood at a distance and eyeballed me. Wherever I went he kept staring at me. I went into the bathroom and he watched. I left the bathroom and he was still staring at me. I walked out of the courthouse and he followed me until I got into the car and drove off. He called me that night, telling me to settle on the original figure offered.

'You'll fucking regret it, Jack. You will be so fucking sorry, you bitch. I will slam you.'

I didn't sleep well at night. It was exhausting – I kept going back and forth in my mind, questioning if it was worth it. Lucky for David I never knew how to record our conversations on my phone.

When I went through the Victorian Family Court system, which runs on a 'no blame' premise, financial abuse had just started to be spoken about in the media. It was a new assertion. Emotional abuse barely made a mention – it often left deeper scars than the physical ones. It's like water torture.

I was advised to attain what was rightfully mine so I could raise Angus by myself, but I knew I would have a fight on my hands. Next we went to a court-appointed psychologist with whom David flirted with the whole time. It was downright embarrassing. She advised the judge that I was to move as close as possible to where David lived as I'd yet to secure a permanent home to live in. I was to have Angus seventy percent of the time and David was allowed the remaining thirty percent. I never understood her reasoning; I had seventy percent but I had to move closer to him!

Eventually a substantial monetary settlement was made at the eleventh hour before we went before our judge for the second time. David had to have been advised by his counsel very clearly that if our case returned to Judge Simpson, it wouldn't look good for him. David sacked his two other barristers for being idiots (his words not mine). What would they know, right?

What was more enjoyable was that, because of his egotistical behaviour it cost him a lot of money, more than necessary. I gladly stood by and watched, knowing that nothing hurt him more than losing money. It sounds odd, but it's those little moments that bring you joy and keep you buoyant and focused.

At Angus' weekly swimming lessons one afternoon, I sat on the sidelines with my girlfriend, Leeanne. I saw Jane coming down the ramp, looking for me.

'What's wrong, Jane? Why are you here?'

'Oh my God, I had to come and tell you something so funny. Rowen's good friend Casey went to a party a couple of weeks ago and she hooked up with David.'

My mouth dropped open. 'So, how was he? … No, don't tell me, I know. He was crap in bed, right?'

She started nodding. 'She said he was really bad, like, *really bad*.'

It was these tiny moments in time that kept me laughing when things became tough. It's the times when you can look back and say to yourself, 'See, he was as bad as I thought. I wasn't crazy'.

The day before a 9 am court appearance, Margo strongly advised David's new legal counsel that she would turn him into the ATO because of his business books. They didn't tally up – something was very wrong. Margo wasn't a forensic accountant but her husband was and he loved his job. It was his passion to numerate. So, after dinner one night, she just happened to ask him his opinion. He came to bed the following morning at 3 am. He'd found the holes. Bless him.

I was standing in the car park of Margo's offices, smoking a cigarette. I'd taken up smoking to replace drinking to help with the stress, which is ridiculous in itself as nicotine is a stimulant, but I needed something. Margo met me outside to give me the news. The email had just arrived – it was over. A settlement had been reached. He'd signed the documents. It may be just a simple act of a pen hitting the paper to make a personable squiggle but it's everything by the law. No signature, no deal.

After eighteen months it was finally done. I gave Margo the biggest hug. She was right all along; she called David 'a goanna in a crocodile suit'. All talk and no action.

I made five calls: Jane, Anne, Scarlett, Clair and Leanne. They were simple calls to relay such good news but I was depleted. To celebrate I went across the road to Kmart and bought Angus three new toys – something I'd never been able to do since he was born. After the financials had been settled, I had to start thinking of how I could start making a proper home for the two of us. I needed to apply for a mortgage to buy a house and that would mean I needed a job – university had to wait. It would have been too much to parent, work and study. The final one had to go on hold for a while.

David agreed verbally to be civil. I knew in my heart that he viewed the court settlement as a huge loss as it cost him so much money, not to mention his ego and his pride. If divorce was a game, then he lost big time. He picked up his bat and ball and went limping home. He was indebted to those who he borrowed money from to fight me. It was the unlosable fight in his eyes –

but he lost. I was then seen as being too low for him to spend emotional time on; now I didn't matter. And compared to a lot of women who go through nasty divorces from their abusive husbands and partners, I knew how lucky I was.

For the sake of Angus, for a few months after court we managed to keep to that agreement, but I should have known it wouldn't last. I have this stupid habit of wanting organised and calm child rearing. In truth, I never thought it was a big ask. I never taunted David about his monetary loss, I knew when to walk away and all I wished was to get on with life. He agreed that we were to respect each other. Respect each other's lives, each other's space. Mine with Angus and he with whomever he chose. In all honesty I truly wanted him to find a partner who deep down he wanted to be with. After seeing that video years previous, I felt in my heart it wasn't a woman he needed to be with to be happy but it wasn't my choice. I didn't care and yet I cared enough that I just wanted him to be happy and then maybe he'd be kinder. Kinder to others but, most importantly, to himself.

He saw Angus every Wednesday night and every second weekend, starting after school on a Friday night. There was no animosity – it was meant to be simple. But his choice in partner backfired with detrimental effects.

2011

I finally found my feet after the divorce became official and left the emergency accommodation. We stayed in a small rental as our new home was built.

I was given the opportunity through Eastern Health to be apart of a course for women who were going through domestic violence; violence we'd experienced through marriage or partnership. It was there that I was to meet our group facilitator, Sophie, a family counsellor who specialised in family violence. The course included discussions on what we had separately been through – some of the group were still living through it. We were then asked to express it into art forms. In week five, when I was on the floor cutting up magazines to make a montage of my life, it dawned on me that I used to be an artist. I'd completely forgotten over the fifteen-year period of so much grief that I was creative; I was astonished that I could draw. It came flooding back. I'd stopped communicating my feelings – it was as if I'd buried everything away – but I was finally able to express myself again.

Art was my expression; an extension of myself, no matter what anyone thought. Even the way I'd dressed over the years with David was an indication of how I felt. I used to be bold and strong in my fashion choices; now thought I felt like nothing, I was empty and tired. I was the definition of beige. Over the years I'd put on a lot of weight due to eating my emotions, my shame. I cut most of my hair off and dyed it brown so no one would even consider looking at me, but, unfortunately, I did catch someone's eye and he wanted to change me.

Just because you've left a painful relationship behind you, it doesn't mean anyone you meet in the future will be any better. You have to keep the red flags in the back of your mind or you could end up in the same situation again. Like me, for example.

Russell was a single father of a daughter and lived alone. He knocked on my door the night I moved into the group of units and told me I had left my car door open and didn't want my battery to go flat. I thought it was very kind of him and left it at that. After a few months of getting to know one another, we then started casually dating. There was no commitment from either of us. Then one day he asked me away on a short holiday. It would just be the two of us and after discussing it with Jane I accepted his offer. I was tired and she said I deserved a break after the past couple of years of living in an extremely volatile and unpredictable marriage. We were going away for two nights as I felt that was long enough to be away from Angus. The thought of heading to a warmer climate was exciting; to be taking a break, where any getaway seemed to me a luxury.

We left Tullamarine Airport and flew north for two hours. I'd like to write that I'd never noticed his behaviour before but he'd been doing things and again I'd been ignoring them. Whilst we were flying a young guy sitting next to me started up a conversation. I could tell Russell was upset I was speaking to someone else. It was just another 'Russell moment', as I liked to call them.

Finally we touched down in sunny Queensland and it was postcard perfect. Collecting our luggage, we headed to our beachside high-rise accommodation in our rental car. The weather was superb, the ocean was calm and I could already feel myself relax even before we officially booked into our room. The sun on my face and the salty air calmed me immediately. The feeling wasn't too last long though.

After we dropped off our bags, Russell decided to drive me around the area and show me some of the sites. Unfortunately, he must have forgotten that some of the side streets were one way only and proceeded to drive up one of them in the wrong direction. Anyone could have made the mistake, but a young guy on a pushbike peddled past our car and decided to yell, 'Mate, you're going the fucking wrong way'.

With that flippant comment paradise was shattered. I had never witnessed Russell in such a state of anger; it was the epitome of road rage in all its glory. He immediately turned the car around and started to chase the kid on the bike, but because we had few cars ahead of us Russell kept on trying to pass them on the pavement. I was hanging on to my seat, screaming at him to stop. He was determined to catch up with this kid, all rationale gone. Finally, the kid cut through a grass-filled park and, to Russell's horror, he disappeared. I was aghast and told him to immediately take me back to the hotel to collect my bags. I was going home on the next flight. I was seriously alarmed by what I'd just witnessed. He apologised and started trying to rationalise why he was upset. He said I was ruining his holiday by not seeing it from his perspective.

I froze, thinking about the situation I was in, what I had put myself in. My first mistake was to feel I had to ignore what had just occurred. It was his shocking behaviour and again my mistake for making excuses for him. I became embarrassed instead of angry. I was repeating my old ways, but instead of fight or flight, I was turning it inwards thinking how I could change the situation instead of standing my ground. Getting out of there was what any sane woman would have done. I didn't have the money to fly home. I sat in a state of feeling ashamed but couldn't do anything about it.

I grew up in a household where my mum was constantly doing that for Dad; no matter how bad his actions became. At least now I could understand that the feeling of unease I was sensing was being acknowledged by me and not dismissed completely. I felt it. I could see it but at the time I couldn't interpret it through affirmative action. Instead, I remained on high alert for the duration of the trip. When I'm on high alert I go into survival mode, agreeing with my aggressor to hopefully keep them calm. I'm highly wired, seriously charged and barely sleep. I have three speeds when I'm overly stressed. They are as follows:

- Manic and vocal.
- Manic with no voice.

Or my favourite …

- Sleep. I curl into a cocoon and lock in my emotions, holding them closely whilst having intense nightmares.

The next morning I watched the sunrise from our fifth-floor apartment, listening to the sound of the rolling surf I stared at the repetitive rolling pace of the water. The sand looked inviting. I hadn't slept properly and was still left feeling over-amplified. A jog along the endless sandy beach would refresh me properly; it had to be a better day, it just had to. My friend the eternal optimist was there to push me through a corrected day. I put on bathers with a pair of shorts and runners, and made my way down to the warming sand. As my jogging picked up pace, I imagined myself becoming more cheerful, happier with each step. An affirmation. I finally arrived back to the front of our apartments forty-five minutes later. I stripped off my shorts and shoes to reveal my bathers, then ran into the surf. I didn't care I didn't have a towel; I'd dry in the sun.

I didn't notice Russell. He'd been waiting on the dunes for me. Joining me in the water, wading deeper, he looked annoyed. Something was upsetting his morning. Again, a feeling of guilt came over me. I dived under, only coming up for air, trying to strip a feeling of fault away.

He said men on the beach were staring at me. 'Cover up as soon as I get out of the water, Jackie. What were you thinking?'

It was humiliating. I wish I had the strength to tell him what I wore was my business and that he had the problem, that he was threatened, but I didn't even try defending myself. Just before you visualise me looking like a Kardashian in a florescent G-string bikini (shit, I wish), I was wearing a navy one-piece Speedo!

Once inside again, he started breakfast, and the conversation changed. Again it was Russell talking. This time it was about his house. This was where he used to live when he was married. He started telling me he was renting it out, as he couldn't afford the mortgage repayments by himself. He then started asking me about the payout I received from my settlement and how I could rent out my home that was being built.

'Russell, why would I want to rent my house out? Angus and I need somewhere to live.'

His banter was exhausting me, his nasally voice grinding. 'Well, I was thinking you could move in with me.' He sounded almost hopeful.

He must have seen the look on my face that I needed more explanation. I couldn't understand where the discussion was going.

'Why? Why would I want to rent out my new home and move in to your tiny rental?' I asked. I was so tired and started becoming short. My polite pretence started to crack.

He calmly stated, with a look of conceit, 'Well, I think it would be an opportunity for us to start anew and I can't think of a better place to start fresh than at my place in Balwyn. Me, you and the kids. We could be an instant family and I could get more time with Emily. She could move back with me. Her mother's a slut.'

Then it hit me why he invited me away; it was my settlement. He miraculously popped onto the scene and was reorganising my financials. It was so transparent it was embarrassing, but I was embarrassed I hadn't seen it sooner. It wasn't me he wanted but my money, as little as it was. It was more than what he had though. He also wanted me to act as his female accomplice in getting his child back. He'd spoken so ill of his ex and when I was exposed to their heated arguments I felt sorry for their daughter. He never picked his times to argue with her either. When they spoke it was always a verbal brawl of who could degrade each other most. Maybe it was deliberate to show me who was the boss, to allow me to see him as an alpha.

I stayed silent, wishing I could disappear, wishing I hadn't accepted his offer to go away. I squinted, put on a fake smile I hoped he wouldn't detect, and closed my eyes. 'I'll have a think about it.'

I was being polite; it was out of fear, fear of not wanting to upset him. I could now see the red flags, but it was too late – for now at least.

That afternoon the weather mimicked my mood. Climatic clouds rolled in as locals warned us that the tail of a hurricane from further up north was about to hit us. They were right, it did – metaphorically too. The weather turned beautiful blue surf into a cappuccino froth that lapped Broadbeach, rolling brown bubble tumbleweeds across the wet sand, drenched by sheets of horizontal rain.

Nothing was good enough for Russell, from when I unpacked my bag and placed my toiletries in the bathroom to how I hung my clothes in the closet. He showed me how he liked his lunch and dinner table to be set, insistent I prepare the meals while he watched. His premise was that I was to learn not to put too much on my dinner plate – I needed to keep my figure in check. When we first met, he told me unreservedly I was too overweight.

I had just come from being married to Mr Control and I wasn't in any condition to be spoken to like a child, but again I stayed quiet. I had endured the wrath of too many men who felt they weren't being heard nor praised for helping a woman 'find her best person'.

So many regrets. If I could have driven a car home I would have done so, there and then, but I couldn't. If I felt I could have called a family member to help get me on a flight back to Melbourne I would have, but I didn't, I'd look like I'd failed again.

'For God's sake, what have you gotten yourself into this time, Jack?' I could hear my sisters as if they were next to me; but it was in my head only, they would have helped me if they knew.

So again I did what I was best at when under intense pressure: I developed one beast of a migraine, threw up in the bathroom and then slept through the second night until the day we were due to fly home on the 7.30 flight from Coolangatta to Tullamarine.

And the surprises didn't stop. While I'd been living in my sleeping cocoon, Russell had braved the weather and went shopping at Pacific Fair, purchasing some dresses he considered acceptable for my body type. As I looked on in disbelief, he explained they would show off my body. 'But they're not too revealing.'

Listening to his babbling again, he had the audacity to ask me to reimburse him. Just when I thought he couldn't do anything worse he asked me to get dressed as he was taking me somewhere special to lunch before we boarded our return flight home. We drove through shocking rain and arrived at Palazzo Versace, where we parked and headlined into their main dining room. I told him before we set foot in the place that I wasn't going to split the bill. He then insisted he'd be paying, with a curt smile. 7.30 EST couldn't come soon enough.

When our drinks arrived he proceeded to hand me a list. It was delivered on a worn, folded piece of off white paper, containing all his wants and must-haves in a woman who he wanted to be in a serous relationship with.

The list read as follows:
(Note: the words in italics are what he wasn't prepared to compromise on.)

What I Like:	What I Don't Like:
Intelligence	Control freaks!
Honesty	
Kind/thoughtful	Dishonesty
Respectful	
Caring	People who lie or manipulate
Attractive	*Selfish people*
Slim	
Active and looks after themselves (Brazil)	Overweight people
Determined	*Not interested in keeping active and fit*
Positive/glass half-full	
Likes wine	*Critical and negative*

And it continued:

> ### What I would want to do with my partner:
>
> - Totally committed
> - Have quality time together
> - Active together – casual run, walking, and keeping fit
> - Go to football, games at the G
> - Travel
> - Share kids and be involved
> - Sex and intimacy – have a happy loving home where everybody counts

If I had my time again, after allowing myself to internally digest the above information, I like to think I would have then said something along the lines of the following:

'Russell, if you don't like control freaks, why are you handing me a list of your likes and dislikes? In fact, why didn't you call your list The Likes and Dislikes of a Control Freak? If you want a kind, thoughtful, respectful and caring partner then I suggest you become a kind, thoughtful, respectful, caring person. If a relationship is going to develop it will happen naturally not via a guidance list.'

When I read 'Active and looks after themselves (Brazil)' my immediate thought was he wanted me to take up soccer to keep fit. Again, I was wrong. He didn't mean the country. He wanted all pubic hair removed from my genital area. He put that on the list. Seriously, who does that? No one in my generation that I knew of. I don't have a 1970s vibe going on, as I believe a little landscaping is good for one's soul, but don't rip out all of the flora. It's not natural. If you attempt to remove all of the garden you could accidentally extract the top surface layer and next thing you know you're fully open to not having anything there to cover something not intended to be so exposed. It's just not a pretty sight in my opinion – but enough talk about vaginas.

Even though Russell spoke about not having an enjoyable holiday in my company as we boarded the plane, he said he felt that we could make this relationship workable. He then requested that I start to think about my own 'list' and email it to him when we returned home.

We finally flew back into Tullamarine at 11 pm, as there had been delays. We caught the shuttle bus to Southern Cross Station and proceeded to make our way on foot with our luggage to collect his car from his work. Just when I thought his behaviour couldn't get any worse, it did.

We were crossing the street near the Melbourne Aquarium to get into Yarra Promenade when a guy in a Porsche decided to run a red light as we were crossing the road. The car wasn't close enough to hit us, but Russell completely lost his shit and threw his carry-on luggage at the already passed car, flinging his clothing over the empty street.

We finally made it to his car. I just wanted to get home to my baby boy and give him the biggest hug I could. When I arrived at Jane's, I slammed the car door behind me. Inside the house I made my way quietly into the room where Angus slept and slid under the covers to be close to him. I was home holding my little boy again; I finally felt safe.

Saturday arrived, two days later, and Russell called. He launched into asking me if I had contemplated my wants and needs for our relationship to move forward. I told him in a tone of voice that I hoped he understood that a relationship between us was not going to work. He sounded hurt but we continued to make small talk and I made the stupid mistake of mentioning that I was taking Angus to a child's play centre to meet Scarlett and her son Ben. I was so happy to be home with my beautiful boy and be a mum again, a role I wouldn't trade for the world. After saying goodbye, I hung up, not thinking any more about it. I breathed a sigh of relief that that was all behind me. On reflection, it should have clicked that I got out of that a bit too easily.

Angus and I were at the packed play centre for a couple of hours. After we left, I decided to drop in on my parents on the way home. We hadn't seen much of each other and I wanted them to see Angus, as I knew they missed him. As Angus was collecting eggs from the chicken coop with Mum, I checked my muted phone and found there were five missed calls from Russell over the two hours I was in the centre. I didn't think anything of it and returned his call without checking the messages he left. If I knew what I was about to expose my ears to, I wouldn't have called back at all.

It was a tone I'd heard before, one that David used to use. Russell sounded so questionable and curious but there was an overtone of pure spite and entitlement. He couldn't cover the anger in his voice; he sounded like he was trying but he couldn't.

I asked why he called; we'd only just spoken earlier. Had he forgotten to tell me something?

'I'm OK, but the question is, Jackie ... are you?' He spat it out.

'Sorry? What do you mean?' I'd always been big at apologising.

In 1988, when hair was big and fluoro was the new black, Nike registered a logo that became world famous, Just Do It. It was then I should have registered the term Just Apologise. I did it constantly, a lot of women do. It's insane – perpetual guilt for no reason. But I digress.

He continued. 'I went to the play centre you told me you were going to and I looked for you and you weren't there! Where were you?'

I automatically started to tell him where I'd been in the centre and why he couldn't find me when it dawned on me that I didn't ask him to join us. He had been checking out where I was without my knowing. Now I was infuriated. It came rolling over me. I'd had a gut full. I verbally launched at him like I'd never done before and I went crazy ballistic at this bastard.

'How dare you fucking follow me!' My rage was evident. I had to walk and hide myself from where Angus was with Mum.

The phone call didn't last that long but it sure as hell went on long enough for him to get the message, or so I thought. I never wanted to see him again. I couldn't have been clearer. I do not mumble – my first language is English, just as his was.

My mother was an English teacher. People often misplaced my birthplace as Belgravia in London due to the way I pronounce my words. I was not born there. I'm Melbourne born and bred. You cannot question my articulation.

This is how articulate I was. 'Stay the fuck away from us you deluded arsehole.' That was delivered in an Australian accent.

Two days later, I eventually calmed down. I received a call from Mum. I was almost cheerful when I picked up her call.

Mum's tone sounded suspicious. 'Hi, Jack. Would you like to tell me what you've been up to?'

I sighed. 'What are you talking about?'

'Well, I just had a delivery from the florist for you and currently there's a bouquet of flowers sitting here in my kitchen that wouldn't look out of place in the Hyatt's ballroom. The delivery guy also handed me a letter addressed to your father and I from the bloke you told to piss off. Russell.' She continued. 'The letter is thanking us for allowing him to be a part of our family and I didn't even know the bloke! What I knew of him I didn't like. What's going on?'

Gritting my teeth and trying to stay composed, I asked her to read out the accompanying card to me.

She read in an overly sweetened tone of voice, 'Dearest Jackie, the most beautiful woman in my eyes and my heart. I love you just the way you are and I miss you! Love, Russell oxox.'

He must have written that he loved me just the way I was in reference to me not wanting to get a Brazilian. He had rebuked on his waxing request!

I could hear Dad in the background laughing. This guy had really pissed me off now.

'Mum, please throw the flowers in the bin.'

'No, Jack. You come and clean up your own mess yourself.'

The line went dead.

After I finished work, I drove over and viewed the bouquet myself. When I saw it my mouth almost hit the floor. It stood in the accompanying ornate glass vase at just under 1.8 metres. The red roses were fanned out and bold. It was huge and greatly accepted by Mum's neighbour Monica, under the positive motto of 'pass it on'. As an added bonus she got to keep the ghastly vase too.

'Are you sure, Jackie? It's too beautiful to just give away like that!'

I put on my broadest smile, showing my all my teeth and my dimples. 'I'm sure, Monica. You are a really kind person – you deserve it. And it doesn't go with my décor anyway. Enjoy.'

I drove back to Jane's. Angus was waiting for me. I told Jane and Andrew what had happened. Andrew offered to have a few words with him, but I had to deal with it myself.

A text message was sent.

> **Russell, you didn't need to send me flowers nor the letter to my folks. Please STOP NOW! Jackie.**

It just wasn't sinking in and I thought it couldn't get any worse.

The following week was hot, so I took Angus over to my parents for a swim. We were splashing about and enjoying the cool of the water. All of a sudden, I saw Mum coming out the back door. She headed quickly in our direction. Remember – she was in her early 80s now so she didn't normally do 'quick'.

'Hurry! Get out. Russell's here!'

'What? Here?' I replied, peering into the glass-walled sunroom. Dad and Russell were having a good old bloke chat.

I went into panic mode. *Stay calm, smile, pretend. Just bullshit your way out of this. Breathe.* I reached out for Angus. He was wearing his green *Ben 10* floaties.

Russell was holding what looked like wrapped boxes. He turned and started walking out through the back door towards us. Angus squealed with delight. Russell had brought over gifts covered in sparkling Christmas paper. Angus splashed, wriggling out of my grip and attempting to dog paddle over to the pool steps. He started getting out, heading closer to the boxes.

'Angus, come back here, sweetheart.'

He didn't listen. What kid would with a blatant enticement like that?

I put on my shiniest, most well-rehearsed fake smile. My only thought was, *Don't make a scene in front of Angus and upset him.*

At this point, most mothers would have launched all the fury they could've mustered at this toxic prick, but from growing up with an abuser I learned automatically to keep calm at all costs. I could never aggravate an abuser; I had to protect my child and myself.

It sounds fanciful but for the following hour I helped unwrap gifts for Angus and played five rounds of *The Hungry Caterpillar* game to get Russell out of my parent's house and to his car.

Once he was leaning on his midnight blue Mercedes, he said he wouldn't leave until I accepted to have dinner with him the following night. With my fake smile and cheeks burning, in a sweet voice I told him that I would have to check my diary and promised to email him in the morning. I waved him goodbye. As he turned the corner, I ran back in the house. I collected Angus and strapped him in the car seat with his new gifts, as he wouldn't let me leave them behind. Mum and Dad thought it was terribly funny; I was beyond scared though. I headed somewhere Russell didn't know of. Clair's parents had offered me their house to sit while they were away on a cruise round Australia. I was thinking that I'd just pop in every second day and water their garden and make sure everything was OK. I had their keys in my handbag so I took up the opportunity that night. We stayed for three weeks, knowing we couldn't be found.

After dropping Angus at childcare one morning, I waited in a side street opposite the units where Russell and I lived. I waited until I saw his car leave for work then I returned to my unit and started pulling all our personal belongings out of the closets and cupboards into large, plastic garden bags. It only took one trip, as we didn't have a lot. The furniture would have to wait until my nephews returned with their Utes the following night. I didn't sleep at all that night and the first person I contacted was Margo to explain what happened. She contacted the estate agent I rented from and they allowed an emergency vacate. Jane contacted our parents to explain the situation wasn't a joke. I couldn't return to the units where Russell lived.

Next person I spoke to was my counsellor, Sophie. I was terrified, left feeling scared and extremely paranoid. She calmly spoke about how I was consciously dealing with it. I just needed to be heard – it was that simple. Instead of reacting I needed to know that I had the confidence to act, to take charge of my life, to protect Angus. I finally decided to send Russell the email that he was waiting for – it wasn't what he was expecting though.

I sent it to his work. I knew that the international company he worked for oversaw all incoming emails. Russell had disclosed to me that in the past he'd been in trouble with his department manager for another email he sent to a work colleague that caused great concern throughout management. It nearly cost him his job. He only needed one more strike and he'd be unemployed. I didn't care anymore. I carbon copied in Anne, Jane, Scarlett and Margo. I wanted him to know his behaviour wasn't hidden anymore. I wanted him to feel embarrassed. I had nothing left to lose.

Subject: Stop Contact

Dear Russell,

Please find this letter to be a formal request to cease contact with either myself, my son Angus, or any of my family members. I understand you think your gesture to me of red roses as well as gifts for Angus was one of being thoughtful but I am finding it imposing on my space, therefore I am asking that you must stop any gifts, letters, emails, phone calls or text messaging immediately. This behaviour feels like stalking to me and is of great concern.

Yours sincerely,

Jacqueline Ellwood

Now, I hear you question if this made him stop. Not immediately. You see, Russell is the type of man who continues to go through life feeling he is always right and has to have the last say. For the sake of continued silence, I let him.

When I read his reply, I had so much adrenaline running through me. My ego wanted to not only answer back but I refrained. Instead, my mind collapsed under a weight of fear and anger at myself for getting into another unavoidable event. I had a faulty radar for choosing people with extreme personality flaws, a homing device for abhorrent men. Instead of focusing my anger on them, I'd turn it on myself. Step by step, I'd retrace my moves, my smile, my look, my speech, the tone of my voice, anything. What did I do to gain the interest of them? I didn't want to victimise myself. It was like begging someone to please show me how to act, how to behave, what to be aware of – anything.

I spent the following months looking over my shoulder, never again wanting to go through such an experience. Would he seek me out again? That was debatable. Once a man of such ego is outed, he normally loses interest – you're beneath him. You've exposed the bully. He'll seek out another woman to control. He will always blame others for his position, carry resentment, and will continue to be critical of others to make himself feel better.

2012 – May

I was in therapy with Sophie again and as our discussion began on my circumstances, I finally got an answer that sat well with me. My heart was so heavy but at least my thoughts became words.

'Why? Why do I continually get drawn to men who are awful? Why didn't my marriage to Charlie work out? I know I was sick but he was a good man, a decent person. He stuck by me and I was repulsed by him. What is wrong with me?' Tears dripped down my face, wetting my shirt.

Sophie looked at me caringly. 'Jackie, you didn't know what a healthy relationship looked like, you still don't. But that's OK. You're acknowledging it and that's a start. You grew up in a home that wasn't safe, wasn't protective, where abuse in all its forms was commonplace, but it was still your world. Somewhere unpredictable was where you felt safe, and you learned techniques to live with it, so it was your normal. Just because you met a decent person who loved you, who you married, who with all his heart said he'd look after you, it didn't guarantee a fit. It wasn't your fault. But hopefully you can now look back and see it for what it was and that's a start, to simply understanding how to get off a path that's so destructive.'

The time had arrived for me to look at all my relationships and pull them apart to try and decipher what I'd partaken in and why. They came in all types too: parents, siblings, friends, work colleagues, partners. I had to learn what made each one function, good and bad. It was up to me to fully understand and notice what red flags were, the bad moves that people played that I played into. Again, it was essential I took responsibility for my moves, not to berate myself but to learn. Sophie and I talked about them for months to come, and that turned into years. There was so much learning to do on my behalf. The patterns with some relationships were so strongly sown that it was like trying to pick and break a woollen thread with a butter knife. It would take time. Mistakes would be made but it was more important I recognise and feel them. I had to learn to sense what wasn't right, and to not feel embarrassed by saying no, and never to apologise for other people's behaviour. I had to learn that I had a voice, and I needed to learn to use it. And that's how I became an advocate for EDVOS and Women's Health East, speaking to groups of people across Victoria and Tasmania about my experiences with domestic and sexual violence. I spoke about the impact of not only the physical and emotional abuse but also the financial and mental health of women and children, and I hadn't even been given a proper mental health diagnosis yet.

To advocate was to be entrusted with something terribly important. To be a voice representing other women in the community who couldn't speak was so rare an opportunity I had to be as clear and concise as possible. Empowerment to me was joining women from all parts of Victoria and learning that I wasn't alone; to be with other likeminded women was to understand their plight too. To hear stories about their past ordeals was truly shocking but by then I'd learned I was more of a help through listening, not speaking over them with a solution. These women didn't want a quick fix from me – that wasn't my role. They needed me to hear them and then through talking with professionals within the field relay a precise message to my audience that we would no longer tolerate the appalling behaviour towards women, children and even family pets. It was as though these men would use their position to abuse anything with a heartbeat. Their time was finally up – they would be exposed and hopefully we'd eradicate domestic and sexual violence completely. I could see it was going to be a very long journey ahead and one too many lives would be lost. I had to grasp that I had a voice and I'd speak, time and again, in front of over one hundred people, both women and men, explaining not only the statistics (which are staggering) but also the personal story I carried. I was one of the faces behind the data, but statistics aren't tangible so we have to stand and face people with real stories of abuse to make it sink in. Then maybe people's eyes will be open to what is happening behind closed doors within their neighbourhood.

I was able to finally verbalise what was happening behind the walls of our homes. I was able to say what my father had done to me, what my husband and boyfriends had done to me. I never spoke their names though; they were now beneath me, not the other way around. I was now confident enough to be able to express to those who didn't understand the ramifications of the abusers themselves and the narcissistic behaviour I or we as a community should no longer be willing to put up with, no longer keeping a secret. If you see it, if you hear it, clearly speak up and expose it for what it is – no excuses.

I'd speak in person to those who were interested in gaining a more personal insight or listen to others who wanted me to hear their stories, at workplaces and community groups. At first I learned from women who went before me, then media professionals who knew the ropes. They would explain the best way to get our stories across, how to make eye contact, how not to be ashamed to speak out. Unfortunately, it even came down to what we wore. I was advised when being interviewed or speaking not to wear anything red; psychologically red is associated with passion, danger and excitement, just to name a few synonyms. It seemed crazy that even though the words coming out of my mouth were insightful, those receiving the information could mentally be focused more on the colour of my lips than the actual message itself. I'd be reminded time and again before giving a talk that all some people would see was the intensity of a hue that would have people judging me and not supporting our cause.

I was interviewed for podcasts and print media across the country and conversed with journalists in my own home for it to be relayed to the public on the evening's news and current affairs programs. It only caused me grief once in the years since I started speaking, occurring at one of my first functions. I was invited to speak in front of local council employees at a breakfast meeting for White Ribbon, a group that started in Ontario in 1991. The White Ribbon campaign is a global movement of men and boys working to end male violence against women and girls. It had a new campaign that was aimed at workplaces to promote respectful relationships and gender equality.

I arrived alongside the Health Promotions and Communications Officer from Woman's Health East, then was introduced to the current Lord Mayor of Monash Council and made very welcome. My adviser Kate spoke first and then I was introduced. I gave a ten-minute talk informing men, who made up the majority of the audience, about my story. It seemed more like an hour of making eye contact with the sea of male eyes. Thankfully I found a small group of females situated in the back corner of the room so I concentrated on them.

Once I'd finished, the group politely applauded. The women I'd focused on stood up, cheering a bit more loudly than normal, obviously understanding my nerves and the message I'd been trying to deliver. All you need as an advocate speaker is the knowledge that maybe someone in the audience understands the message without sounding preachy. I could never lose the feeling though, no matter how often I spoke to live audiences – I'd wonder how many men that I looked out to were abusers themselves. How many of them finished their day by cheerfully farewelling their work colleagues, getting in their car and returning home to a wife and family they'd treat like shit behind closed doors?

I thanked them and made my way to the back of the room where Kate was standing. The Lord Mayor stood up and returned to the podium, where he excitedly mentioned to me the men at the council had partaken in making a video clip for White Ribbon Day. We all looked towards the large screen at the front of the room and it began. Every male who worked for Monash Council came up on a pre-recorded message, staring into the camera, their faces in full view. Speaking clearly, all said the White Ribbon official tag of 'I swear'.

'I swear never to commit, excuse or remain silent about violence against women. This is my oath.'

Then it continued, over and over again, a different face, a different voice, each time with conviction.

I swear.
I swear.
I swear.

The video must have gone only for a minute, but it was too much. I started to hyperventilate. I turned to Kate. She could see the distress on my face and she put her arms round my back and gently guided me outside, away from anyone who could see me. She was at a loss as to what had happened and I couldn't catch my breath. I was sobbing. A lady from the group came to help as well. It took me a while to compose myself and explain what had happened as it took me by surprise too. But I was finally able to let them know. Kate was so attentive and worried.

'Jackie, what happened? You spoke so well. What happened?'

I couldn't believe it; I'd just remembered what they said.

'Each one of them said it. All of them.' I was dumbfounded. 'They all said I swear. I swear, Jackie, I swear I'll never do it again. They all said it. They said they'd never do it again. Since I can remember, Dad said to Mum, "I swear I'll never hit her again". David said it too. But they did.'

I remember my nose running and I was trying to compose myself. I was in public but I just needed time to process it. I was obviously so good at putting on a poker face that I was back with the group and fully composed to answer questions within half an hour.

Once away from the chambers, I was able to sit in a nearby restaurant with Kate for a debrief. I was exhausted again, completely washed out. It triggered something in me that I'd completely forgotten about. It happens at times when advocates who have been through domestic or sexual violence are talking with people. It only takes a small, forgotten prompt to ignite something you had put away in memories long gone.

When speaking in front of a large audience of health care academics from universities across Australia at Population Health Congress 2015 in Hobart, it happened again. Something popped up out of nowhere. Once the lecture had finished and I was making my way to the back of the room, an older gentleman stood up and put both his hands on my arms. He was enthusiastically thanking me for sharing my story, but I immediately pulled back out of fear; I couldn't believe he launched at me. The women sitting round him stood up and grabbed him, telling him to sit down. I'm pretty sure he got the message, as he was very apologetic. Note: maybe I should have warned people never to touch me when I'd been speaking about abuse. It doesn't gel well! Each time I spoke, what happened to me was always in the back of my mind. To have a man come towards me so unexpectedly spooked me terribly, but again I got over it.

I'm not the type of speaker who can just read off my notes without a connection; it's not a performance. The focus is to speak as clearly as possible so the audience can understand the implications of what abuse does to a woman, a teenager or child from all socioeconomic backgrounds, from all homes across Australia.

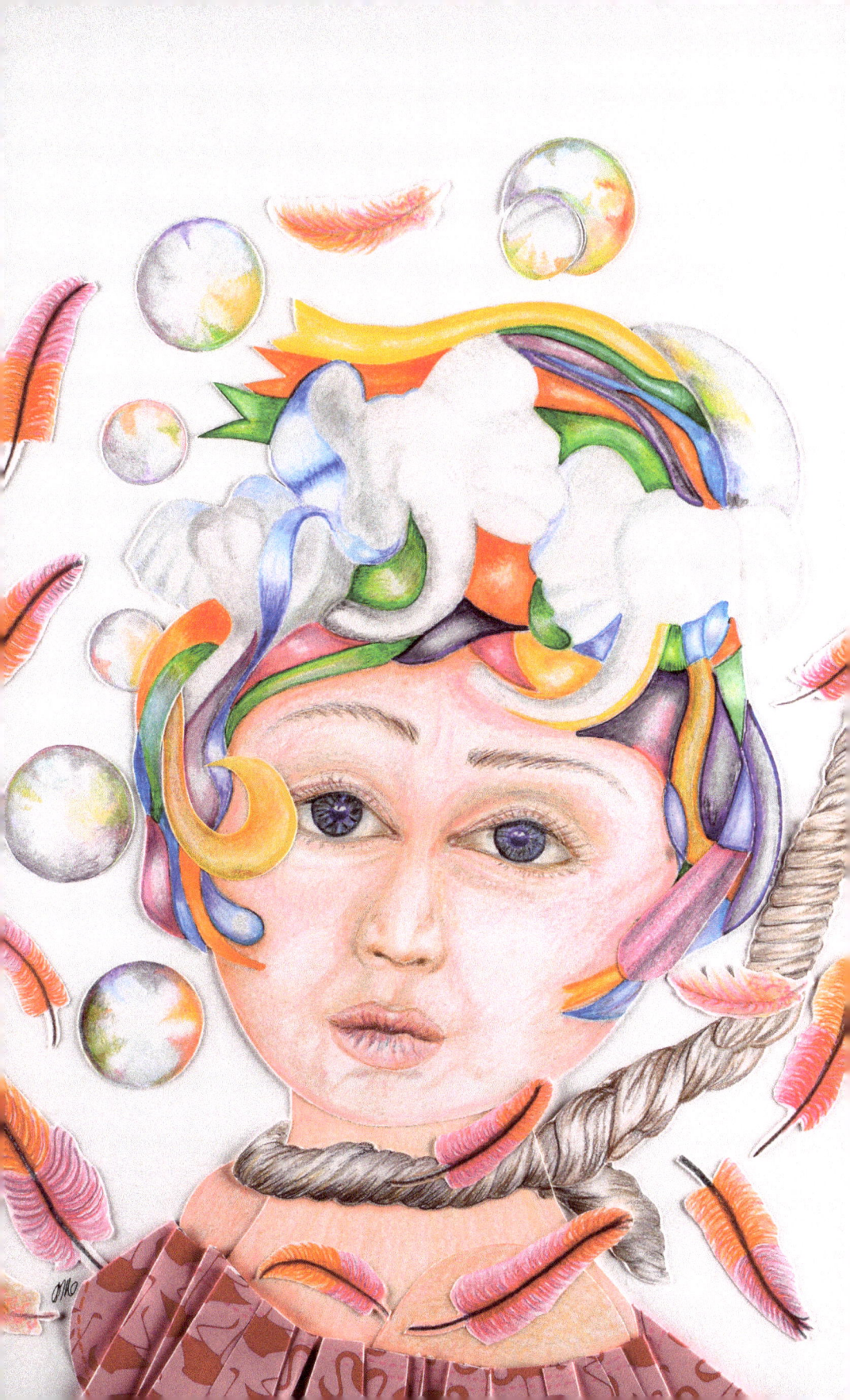

2012 – July

I was back living at my parents' house again, on the verge of another hypomanic episode. Whenever these occurred my family knew that all I asked was that Angus be looked after and protected. Dad would collect Angus after school and he and Mum would care for him until I was well enough.

I stayed up for days with little sleep. Over three nights, a few broken hours of sleep at most – that's when the psychosis began. Walking to the bathroom, I nervously sat on the toilet because I thought I'd fall in. I looked down at the tiled floor. In unison all of them lifted off the ground and flipped over, not unlike a physical domino effect. Over and over, they'd tumble, each time changing to a different colour.

I spent a couple of days landscaping my parents' huge front yard, digging holes for no apparent reason. I'd strenuously push large rocks back and forth into no place special. I attacked overhung trees with loppers, pruned roses that looked uneven, knelt and pulled out stubborn weeds that had been tap rooted for years. The harder they were to remove, the more aggressive I became to rip them out. My hands started to bleed and swell from the punishment I put them through.

I never ate; there wasn't time to refuel and I certainly wasn't hungry. As night-time fell, I'd be rummaging through Mum's sewing room, looking for anything to create. I'd cut faces out of cardboard; I was obsessed with drawing faces of women, I called them my little Ninbin Nymphs. My brushes were loaded with watercolour paint, fine-tipped Italian ink pens portraying full lips, eyes of every hue, eyebrows and piecings. Dyed wool would be strewn out and plaited to become hair. Buttons became earrings. Face after face I'd produce, over and over. Once completed, I would go out into the garden's darkness with a torch I'd found in the kitchen. I'd squat, seeking out twigs and leaves, gently sorting through them. It was a mission to pick the best shapes and sizes before the snails found them, leaving their slimy path distributed across the foliage.

The face masks accumulated more and more, all spread out in the sunroom floor into first light. My favourite part was hearing the birds waking up. I recall hating the thought of anyone interrupting me, especially Mum; I never wanted anyone ruining my racing one-track mind.

In the past Angus had asked me, 'Mummy why don't you make faces of boys instead of girls?'

It was because girls were safe; girls were diverse and beautiful. They had so many features about them that I loved. I saw men as hard in feature, wrong, never truthful, invasive, entitled.

'I don't know how to draw a boy. I wouldn't draw a boy unless it was you, and I wouldn't do it any justice because to me you're perfect.'

I'd kiss him and he'd run off.

I was refusing to see another psychiatrist, even a doctor. I'd ignore Mum's requests and walk off. She stopped trying. Dad kept his distance but also kept quiet – that's all I wanted. He saw me as unpredictable and didn't know how to deal with me so he stayed away. I didn't want him anywhere near me, but Mum was different. She'd seen me in this state before, but it still wasn't easy for her. She was in her early 80s now. Her role had changed into protector and pacifier but she was exhausted.

Suddenly things started to disappear from around the house. Anne had come over and warned Mum that I could try and take my life again. Peroxide that had been in the bathroom cupboard from long ago vanished – she thought I'd drink it. Sharp objects including pens and a letter opener that used to be near the phone, suddenly gone. The garage was to be locked in case I found ropes Dad had collected over the years, as well as any cutting instruments. The cars were left out on the driveway, homeless. Mum just didn't know what to do with me; she knew I was high but she waited for the drop. She prayed it would be sooner than later.

But the delusional mania was to continue for a little while longer. Walking past a large wicker basket my parents kept their old newspapers in I locked onto an image of an elderly woman from India who was a street beggar. I immediately felt we had a connection, this woman and I – I read her thoughts. I became so distressed about her suffering, her being so poor, a non-existent in society, an untouchable. Mum came running. The woman was living on the street because she'd lost both her legs but nobody wanted her, not even her family. After the distress a huge wave of calm came over me, easing the anxiety. I could finally see her for what she was – a beautiful soul. It was as if the sky opened up revealing the Milky Way on a crystal clear night. She was at peace with it now. I started sobbing because who was I to question her position in society? She'd told me so: she was a spirit on Earth, wise beyond anybody I'd ever come across. I wasn't allowed to pity her. Now I was angry and panicked, as though I had to protect her from being judged.

'Don't pity her, Mum. Don't you pity her. She doesn't like that.' I kept repeating it. 'Stop it, don't.'

'Jackie, stop.' Mum was looking at my hands; she took them in hers. 'Just stop.' She shook me. 'Please just stop.'

My fingers were covered in blood; it was under my nails, clogged skin from scraping my scalp. Bloodletting released the pressure – relief came.

I ran up to the bathroom and I was over the sink, heaving. I wanted to vomit and that's when God spoke to me.

'Jackie, you will be all right.'

I stopped and looked around. I didn't know the voice but it was simple and strong, yet soothing. Every word was pronounced and spaced so clearly. I turned to see Dad but he wasn't there. Mum either. I was alone. I don't remember how long I stood in the room but I knew someone spoke to me. I then felt calm. It was definitely God.

It was then time to descend; I needed to sleep.

I was in bed, with Mum sitting close to me. I was panicked, rocking.

'I can't sleep, I can't sleep.'

Scared to sleep, I was overly tired from not having slept for days. It was too much – now I could feel the madness taking over me.

Mum started rubbing my back, as she did when I was little, to soothe me. There was a pattern she followed. Always her right hand, she twisted to suit the movement, not wanting to disturb her pattern arrangement. The palm of her hand facing down on my back, the hold gently anchored her movement so only her fingers moved like soldiers in unison. Her fingers would lift and start gently patting me, then her whole hand would move in an anti-clockwise motion, calming my panic; a firm pat, pat, pat. Repeat. Pat, pat, pat. Repeat. Sleep came only after a few false starts. Just when she thought I'd fallen into slumber she tried to leave and I'd rise up again ready to leave the bed. She'd return, allowing me more time to settle. And then I slept. Her child just wouldn't sleep.

A dream came to me, so clearly. This time I had a visit from my dear friend Leanne. She was surrounded in white flowers. She spoke to me. She had short, bleached blonde hair, a made-up face, red lipstick. Her voice was husky and smooth. She faced me, looking concerned. 'I need to talk to you.'

'What?'

It was wonderful seeing her.

'Jack, I need to talk to you, but I can't.'

'I'm here, Leanne, just tell me.'

She kept telling me she needed to tell me something, then she turned and walked off. I didn't want her to go. I always loved being in her company. She was full of energy, larger than life.

When I woke up the next day it wasn't until 3 pm when I walked into the kitchen. There were two nurses chatting with Mum at the dining table; the CAT team was kind enough to enter my life again.

'Hi, Jackie. How are you feeling?' They introduced themselves. 'We'd like to have a chat, if that's OK.'

I didn't think I had a choice; I didn't feel like arguing or walking away. After my episode, I was so wasted, burnt out. I hadn't showered in days. I was dirty from wandering around the garden, looking for sticks in the moonlight. Blood was still under my nails from scratching my scalp. I surrendered. The team stayed for an hour and a half, just long enough to meet

Angus and check on his welfare. It was part of their job. My beautiful boy was none the wiser.

Penny, one of the nurses, told me that Mum didn't want me admitted to the local psych hospital. They were convinced that Angus and I were safe, but they'd organised a meeting at 8.30 am the next morning to meet a new psychiatrist.

No trouble. I'll go to tick the box and make everyone happy. Just smile and nod; then I can go back to bed and sleep again.

'Jacqueline, it would be best if you go have a shower. If you need help one of us can assist you. Your mum looks tired.'

Everyone was smiling and nodding.

'No, I'm good.'

Mum helped me after they left. Feeling warm water running over my skin was intense as I become overly sensitive to feeling when manic. The water was warm but felt like it was effervescent; I remember laughing because it tickled. Crazy.

After, Angus hugged my legs.

'I love you, baby boy.' I kissed him on top of his head. This time I was in clean clothes, feeling fresher but still tired. 'Nanny said you can help cook dinner. Would you like to do that? Mummy has to go and have a rest again.' I returned to bed, but this time sleep came, as I was feeling calmer after being given Diazepam.

Leanne was there again, framed in white flowers. 'I need to talk to you.'

'Then tell me,' I said.

'I can't.'

I was hopeful in asking, 'Can I call you?'

'You can't call me.'

'I can.'

'No.' She turned away and walked off.

Mum woke me. I needed to get up as she was driving me to meet the new psychiatrist. Dad was taking Angus to school. I was in a fog but understood what I had to do. I got dressed.

I don't recall the half an hour trip as Mum gave me another small tablet of Diazepam from the small quantity the nurses had left me, settling my mind. Once we parked, she came around and opened my door, then, linking her arm in mine, we walked to my new doctor's suite. We checked into reception, waited until I was called. He came out of his office and then introduced himself softly by his first name.

'Hello, Jackie. My name is Martyn.'

With Mum's prompting, I followed him into his room. He asked if I wanted her to join us but I knew he was going to ask me questions that I wasn't prepared to share with her. Finally, I was sitting in a comfortable, leather beige chair opposite him. The walls were covered in framed degrees from Melbourne University. So many letters after his name.

He was very polite. 'Thanks for coming to see me today. I understand you're very tired but I'd like to have a chat with you this morning if you don't mind. I'd like to learn a little about you. If you can tell me what's been happening.'

'I'm tired. Too much has happened.' I sat there blankly.

'OK, I'm going to ask you some questions and I just need you, if possible, to answer them. Let's start with medication, drugs. I know it's not easy but I want to help you.'

I nodded. We began.

'You have a son, and his name is Angus.' He was reading off some notes.

'Yes, I'm a single mum.'

'Do you drink?'

Was that a trick question? 'Yes, and before you ask, it's too much.'

He smiled and nodded. 'Smoke cigarettes or anything else?'

'Yes, I smoke cigarettes.'

'Do you take any recreational drugs? Marijuana, cocaine, ecstasy, meth – anything?

'No.' I shook my head.

And then came the question I was dreading. 'My notes say you're not on any medication apart from Diazepam currently to sedate you, and you have been on antidepressants. Can you tell me what you've been given in the past?'

I put my hand on my temple and exhaled. 'I have been on so many drugs since I was 26 that I've lost count. I've had so many doctors, psychiatrists. I wouldn't know where to go for the information you're wanting. I know it's a lot.'

'That's OK.' He took in a quick breath. It sounded like his train of thinking was pivoting in another direction. 'I'm going to mention some drugs, you tell me if you've had them.' He reached for his Monthly Index of Medical Specialities then started.

I nodded; I'd try.

We stared piecing together a list, but only got halfway when my time was up. I was too tired to continue anyway. I returned the following morning at the same time. Dad drove. He asked if I wanted him to accompany me as Mum did but I said no. I was feeling well enough to go on my own. He stayed in the car reading the *Herald Sun*.

Back sitting in front of Martyn again, we returned to discussing medication, reaching twenty-one different names. It was then I opened up more about my history. He was poised to take notes.

'Tell me about your life as a whole. Is there anything that happened or you felt that was a big event, or a strong feeling you've had? To put it simply: who is Jackie?'

I started. It began with the abuse from Dad, what he did to Alex and I, then my behaviour as a young adult. The drinking, stealing from my father, the spending, the ecstasy I felt when I spent money on others. My hyped behaviour at times, the lows afterwards. The extreme paranoia for no reason. Feelings of grandeur. My two marriages, my two divorces. My attempted suicide, admission to Belmont Hospital, ECT, Banksia Hospital with postnatal depression – all personal failures. The abuse from David and another partners. The sexual assault when at uni. There was no organisation of events that occurred. My wanting to become a sex worker.

'So, did you?'

'No, I didn't.' I shook my head in disbelief at how close I felt I got. 'My sister Jane stepped in. Only her and her husband know.'

'Was that something you'd always planned to do?' he asked, but wasn't judgemental in his questioning.

'No, it was the thrill and at that moment it just made sense. My thinking was erratic, I know that, but my thought seemed logical.' I shook my head over it. 'I've never been someone who could pick up or have a one-night stand; it just sounds wrong to me. I remember what Dad said when I was really young – I'd be a slut if I slept around – so I never had casual sex or "slept around" like a man would, what he'd get away with. I want to say it was because I needed the money but it wasn't, though it would have been a lot for me. It was this enormous need for sex. It was an overwhelming feeling since I was young, very young. I don't know why saying it feels so wrong, but it wasn't then.' I was so ashamed and I was looking to offload the weight I had on my shoulders. I continued trying to explain my rationale. 'If someone paid me for sex then there be no expectation, would there? I enjoy sex, but I didn't want any chance of something coming of it. I'm not good at it – relationships. To have a transaction with someone who I never had to explain myself to – just let me have sex with someone and then leave me to my own life, to raise my son. It's so illogical and wrong when I bring Angus into the picture; but then I never thought of him when I felt high.' I stopped, waiting to see his disgust at my reflection. I was crying now.

'It's OK. You don't have to apologise.'

I continued. 'I think too I just wanted to have someone touch me. I had to be in control though; I couldn't stand the idea of being with anyone where a relationship developed. I'm not good at that – two marriages. Each time I fuck up I have to wipe the slate clean and start again. Angus was the only good thing that happened. That was the best thing I've ever done, becoming a mum. He's everything to me.'

'Do you consider yourself a perfectionist?' he asked

'It's more like looking back at the huge mess I've made and I have to try again next time even harder but something happens again. It might be a small stuff up but I've ruined it. I get so paranoid that everyone is angry with me, talking about me. I can't deal with it so I just walk away. It's same with the number of jobs I've had – so many. I was offered so much; my career was set but I pissed it all away.'

'So you studied merchandising, art and photography at RMIT. You're gifted in that area, you're creative.' He raised his eyebrows and smiled in acknowledgement.

I nodded. All I saw was someone trying to think.

'OK.' He stopped again. 'When you go into a depressive state how long will it last for on average?'

'It could be a few weeks. It's horrible, I feel like dying. I just don't want to be here anymore.'

'And Angus? Do you ever have feelings of harming him?'

I was horrified at him asking me that. 'Never. I would never touch him. He's my world. It's just me – like he'd be better off without me being his mum.'

'Now with this last episode you said you heard a voice – you say God. Did you see God?'

'No, I only heard him, but really clearly.' I could feel Martyn's train of thought. 'And the floor tiles moved, they flipped over, changing colours. When I first had a breakdown, I thought I saw a woman on the end of my bed. I think it was my grandmother but it wasn't her face, it was an elderly woman, but she was just looking over me, as a comfort.'

'We call that a visual hallucination.' He kept writing notes.

I thought I'd spilled my guts to someone again who, like all the other shrinks, didn't have a clue what was wrong.

He spoke so quietly and controlled. 'Jackie, I feel you've definitely been misdiagnosed over the years.'

I waited. I felt at the mercy of someone who might have the answer to why I was faulty.

'You have what's called bipolar. I'm not sure if you know of it.'

'I saw a psychiatrist in Banksia Hospital when I was there after I had Angus. She thought that, but only briefly, then changed her mind. She changed her diagnosis to postnatal depression.'

'I'm sure you did have postnatal depression but you have bipolar 2. It's not any less than being bipolar 1 – it's really a number to differentiate it.'

I remember quietly whispering in reply, deadpan and empty. I was drained of energy again. 'That's definitely me; I'm different.

'So, I'm going to try you on some new medication. Now, when you were at Belmont the psychiatrist there gave you lithium, which didn't work.' He was thinking out loud again. 'I'm going to try two new medications together. One you'll take at night. This will allow you to get some rest, a proper sleep. The next you will take twice a day. If you look it up online, it's actually used as an anticonvulsant for people with epilepsy. I'll print you out an information sheet on it.'

Now I was confused. 'But I'm not an epileptic, am I?'

'No, you're not, but for some reason – and we don't know why yet – it works. Some medications are used on people for different reasons than what they were made for originally. You will feel the full effects in about two weeks.'

'I'm quite sensitive to things, medication in the past, allergies to food, smells – it becomes overwhelming at times.'

'OK, it could be sooner then.' He was nodding. He went on to explain the adverse effects. In case anything showed up, I was to call him immediately.

With the scripts in my hand, he walked me to reception and made another appointment for a week's time.

'Call me immediately if you're not feeling well. I'll contact CAT and let them know where we're at so you can call them. They have a twenty-four-hour team for after normal business hours.' He smiled. 'Take care.'

To say I was bewildered would not be an exaggeration. Apart from simple greetings, Dad and I drove home in silence; I needed to process what had happened. Either this wasn't going to work like everything else I'd tried and I'd be back to square one or it would work. I needed to decide whether or not to drop the scripts in; it was almost an apprehension. I didn't want to be disappointed again and left upset. But what if he was right? I needed to read up about bipolar 2. I'd heard of bipolar but I didn't know there were two types. I didn't want to tell anyone yet.

Once home I walked down the street and put the scripts in to our local chemist. Martyn said one of them would allow me to sleep correctly. I got both medications. I'd decide if I'd take both after dinner.

Reading the information printout he'd given me about contraindications, it didn't sound good. I explained to Mum I was going to take some new medication but I didn't explain what it was for. It wasn't only myself who would feel let down if I was to go backwards again. I also told her about the side effects, including sleeping more solidly, in case Angus woke during the night. It was rare if ever it happened. He could have a fighter jet flying around his bedroom and he still wouldn't wake.

After dinner I took a shower and spent time with Angus before our nightly routine of brushing our teeth. Then I read him three books. Angus went to sleep as we quietly spoke about his day. Once he was asleep, I returned to the bathroom and took the pills. I went to bed and slept, dreaming again.

Leanne was framed in white flowers. 'I need to talk to you.'

'You can. What is it?' I said.

'No, I can't talk.'

'Can I call you?'

'You can't call me.'

'Yes, I can.'

'You can't.'

2012 – July

Five days. That's all it took.

I remember the exact moment: I was sitting on the lounge room floor with Angus, playing snap with colourful cards. Something changed, a switch, a light bulb on in my brain. It was as though I could mentally sense more clearly. A calm came over me. It felt like pure logic, it was rational. I felt at peace. I had never felt like that, ever. Not high, not low – just rational.

I left it another forty-eight hours before I told anyone. I had to test it.

Angus was staying with David that night so I decided to tell Mum and Dad straight after dinner before they drank too much. I'd printed out some information so they could read about it and understand it.

'Um … I have something to tell you,' I told them.

They waited, staring at me.

'Martyn – Dr Lyndhurst – the psychiatrist I've been seeing … '

They looked very calm yet wide-eyed. They actually looked really tired.

'He's diagnosed me. He thinks I have bipolar 2.'

They both nodded their heads. No statement, no disagreement. No yelling – nothing.

'Here's a printout if you'd like to read about it. I needed to read about it; it might help you understand.'

Mum then asked, 'Are you taking all the medications he prescribed?'

'Yes.'

'Excellent, keep it up. We love you. We just want you better.'

And that was a huge let down; they acted like they knew what was wrong. I was stunned. I wasn't expecting a brass band, or even confetti and streamers, but something would have been nice. I then called Jane, and Anne. Again, they weren't surprised.

I rang Clair and Scarlett; it was the same reaction. They were all acknowledging it but it was as though they knew it. I didn't know it; how could they have known it? This was the biggest thing that had ever happened to me but they were behaving as though they were in on the secret. I then tried to call Leanne again but had to leave a message.

Jane came to visit me a few days later, the night before Angus and I were to head home.

'I want to have a chat. First off, Andrew and I are so happy that this medication is staring to make you feel better. It's been a long time coming, too long,' she said.

'I'm scared how people will see me having gotten a proper diagnosis, but I feel so much better. I've never felt like this before,' I said.

I didn't know anyone with bipolar. I was so comfortable with the way I felt, but apprehensive too. I wanted to continue feeling well but I was scared of being judged.

'We want to ask you something. We've bought a block of land close by and we were wondering if you would like to put your home on the market and build a new home on it with us. We're thinking three separate units. I have the plans here.' She presented me with drafted plans of three buildings positioned on a plot of land. She continued to talk about how she'd own two of the units and I'd make up the third. It was a spacious two-bedroom unit with a garden all of my own. I immediately loved the idea. It felt right. Angus and I had the opportunity to start afresh. We would live next door to Jane. It would suit us brilliantly. If I happened to get sick again, she said I needed to be close, as Mum was getting too old. I agreed.

That night I went to bed so happy that we had something so special to look forward to: a new home, a new start. It was perfect.

Again, Leeanne came to me in my dreams. This time, I woke up, crying. Something was very wrong; I felt it.

I went to breakfast with Angus the next day. As he headed off to school with Dad, I explained my dream to Mum.

'The dreams are becoming stronger. Something bad has happened.'

'Honey, it's probably the new medication playing tricks on your mind. Have you tried calling her?'

'Yes, but there's no answer. I've left messages – nothing. I don't even know how to contact her parents. This has been going on for weeks now, and this dream never changes no matter what my state of mind.'

I then took a chance by calling a local funeral home near to where Leeanne lived. For privacy reasons they couldn't confirm if they had held a ceremony for a Leeanne Hensley but I was allowed to leave my details should someone need to contact me. The following day I drove down to her new home on the Mornington Peninsula. No one was home, so I pushed a written note under her door as well as a copy in her letterbox. I just needed to hear her voice.

Heading home I received a call. It was Leanne's dad.

'Jackie, we've never met but I've been looking for you. Leanne passed away three weeks ago.' He sounded so wounded. 'She made you executor of her will. How did you know to look for me?'

'Mr Hensley, I'm so very sorry. I really can't explain it … Leeanne came to me in a dream, over many nights. She told me herself.'

I was astonished that he'd contacted me. I shook with the pure grief that overcame me. In that moment, I felt Leeanne leave me. Even though our time together was brief, I loved her. We had an amazing bond and I think about her every day.

2015 – March

It came time for Angus and I to move into our newly built home – our second – and it couldn't have come soon enough. There had been major positive changes occurring and the move into our second new home went brilliantly. We jointly celebrated Angus' seventh birthday and the housewarming surrounded by family and friends.

I started a new job as manager for a local building company and to be able to provide for our tiny family was the best thing I could have asked for. I felt stronger. I was more confident and was holding down a good job that allowed me to meet challenges head on without overwhelming myself. Life had finally fallen into place. I could finally acknowledge that things were good, but being grateful in the knowledge that it could all fall apart if I didn't look after myself sat on my shoulder as a reminder.

I was receiving a wage and a small amount from Centrelink, as well as David's 120 dollars a month in child maintenance, but I didn't make enough to provide for both of us solely. As David owned a business and dealt in a lot of cash transactions, it was 'confirmed' through his tax records that he only earned 14,000 dollars, which was the benchmark for the most monies that can be earned before you hit the high threshold of supporting any child/or children. His actual earnings were over 120,000 dollars and the house I'd once lived in was last valued at 1.3 million five years previously. The Melbourne market was increasing in value constantly.

In frustration, I contacted Child Support on three occasions and explained my situation but the process was so drawn-out and tedious, as with anything to do with bureaucracy. The hoops I would've had to jump through to prove the father of my child was rigging the system were too many. In the end I settled on the knowledge that I was doing the right thing by Angus and David wasn't – it was that simple. He was a bludger. And in a years' time it was to hit a bigger hurdle – the lowest point possible.

But then I took comfort in the simple things. Both Angus and I were healthy, I was able to work five days a week, making enough money to pay off our mortgage, food, clothes and the occasional outings for Angus, without support from family. I had the capacity to mentally and physically help with homework because my sleep pattern was regular. I could care for my child rather than rely on family assistance. I felt truly fortunate that life was safe, regular, orderly and full of love.

I perceived that David had changed for the better. We were oil and water – we just repelled one another. He had a new partner in his life and I felt she had a positive effect on him. He recently seemed calmer and not disagreeable all the time, but like all things too good, it started to dwindle again.

David's partner's name was Olivia and she was a single mother to a young girl named Anouk who was two years older than Angus. To begin with he was so excited that his dad had a new person in his life and before long we both got a surprise I never saw coming.

One sunny morning I dropped Angus off at David's. I asked Angus for a kiss goodbye when, all of a sudden, Anouk spoke up and said, 'Mum's having a baby.'

I looked at David, surprised, and he sheepishly smiled and confirmed it was true.

'Olivia wanted a baby before she got too old!'

He was going to be a father again. I was shocked but I immediately thought how wonderful it was that Angus was going to have a sibling. He'd be a big brother. I genuinely congratulated David. As I drove off a tear streaked down my cheek and the feeling hit me. I wasn't going to give Angus a brother or sister. I wouldn't have any more children. I never wanted any more kids but it still hurt and took me back to that picket fence dream. It truly had always just been a mirage. Once home I regained my composure and knocked on Jane's door to share the news. We both agreed it was lovely for Angus to have a sibling.

Jane and Clair had been telling me over and again it was time to move on with my life and this was the sign I needed. It felt as though I was heading in the right direction to really move on with my life.

'Jack, you need to jump back on the horse,' Jane said and she was right. So I did.

It had been a while since I had considered having a partner again. I had dated briefly for nine months but it ended amicably and things were going so well I didn't want it to be interrupted. I'd been on a few casual dates but nothing clicked, and then I became so terribly disheartened when I met a new guy online.

I met up for dinner with Todd, a local father of three, and he seemed nice enough but something wasn't right. It felt off, so I decided to finish my meal, wish him the best and be on my way. Unfortunately, he 'forgot' his wallet so I paid the 140 dollar bill. Trying to be optimistic, I saw it as taking the hit to get the arsehole out of my life. Did it work? No.

The next morning at my desk I begrudgingly took a call from him. I got straight to the point.

'Hi, Todd. I really don't want to go out with you again. It won't work out.'

I was silent to let him speak. All I could pick up was the muffled noise of something – I wasn't sure what though. Then he started speaking.

'I … had … a … really … good … time. It … was … so … fucking … good.'

'I beg your pardon?'

Then he let out a cry and the penny dropped. I realised what he'd just done. The cockroach had just ended his masturbation session and had climaxed, feeling, most likely, semen all over his hand and upper thighs. All I felt was an infuriating mix of shock and then anger. I hung up on him and blocked his number on my phone. I closed the online dating account – the four letters of the site expressed my feelings about it: Romance Sucks Very Plainly.

Again, I encountered a stark example of a man needing to control the narrative, and for a while he held it. After the anger died down came embarrassment and hurt. I was left looking over my shoulder for another predator – that's what he was until I finally came to terms in my mind that he was just a bored, certified prick. The worst part of it was that he was a coach of the local girls under 16s basketball team, which his daughter was a team member of. He was a paid supporter of the local footy club, a true local champion. I wasn't the first nor would I be the last woman he would do this to. I could only hope karma would intervene eventually. It was the same story as always though, and if I were to get him angry then he'd give me further grief. I didn't go to the police and have him charged – he didn't even get a warning. I had a history of mental illness and low self-esteem from putting up with too many offenders of all levels, so who would believe me? In my mind, I had dealt with men's poor behaviour in my way. It was safe for me to do it my way – it was my survival method. Too many men got away with too much and I felt that would never change, and that was the truth.

My simple theory stems from growing up with a father who abused me but who was seen as a pillar of the community; no one saw my father in a bad light ever. So who would believe me? I had been married to a man who lied everyday to control his image – he was seen as a brilliant businessman. He came away from the family court looking like butter wouldn't melt, nor was he paying for his son. David got away with so much. So who would believe me?

Once the weekend had started and Angus was with his dad again, Jane allowed me one day to feel depressed over the cockroach issue and then she came over with a bottle of wine telling me my time was up. I actually loved the new depression timeline she had assigned – she had a true gift of organising people. I wasn't to spend another minute allowing a complete stranger to rule my thinking, and she was right.

She said, 'Don't let some perverted dickhead ruin your chance of finding someone, Jack. You deserve to be happy, and even if you don't find anyone, you can't let it stop you from meeting decent people full stop. They do exist.'

While Jane's encouragement buoyed me, the situation with David was just beginning. David's partner, Olivia, had just given birth to a boy, Sam, and Angus was in love with his brother. He couldn't stop talking about him and was even asking to spend more time over at David's to be with the baby, but there was a turnaround not long after.

I was driving home from work one afternoon when I got a call from David. He was terribly upset and proceeded to tell me I had to collect Angus immediately as he had tried to suffocate the baby.

'What? What do you mean?' I was shocked.

He was agitated. 'I'm meant to be working, Jack, and Liv called me home telling me that Angus tried to suffocate the baby with a pillow. She left him in the same room as Sam as she was cooking in the kitchen and she put her head round to check on the kids and Angus had put a pillow on the baby's face. Angus was suffocating my son. Come pick him up now,' he demanded.

2015 – May

I was shocked. David had to be mistaken. Olivia had to be mistaken. Angus would never do that. He loved Sam. I knew my child and Angus didn't have a nasty bone in his body.

I drove to their home and collected Angus. He'd been crying. I picked him up and held him close. I clipped him into his chair and we started our trip home.

'Where are we going, Mum? Why am I leaving Daddy's? Livvy smacked me. What did I do?' He was crying again and looked confused.

I pulled the car over, put on the park break and hazard lights. I hopped in the back seat and just held him. He was sobbing now. 'What did I do?'

He either didn't do anything (which was my bet) or didn't know what he'd done. I was shocked. As soon as I got home, I called Jane into the house when I'd settled Angus to sleep. I just couldn't make sense of it.

'Are you kidding me, Jack? Angus wouldn't hurt a fly, let alone his baby brother. David's insane, and so is that woman he's with.'

'Shh, he'll hear you! What am I going to do?'

'Firstly, document everything. Something's very wrong.'

I couldn't believe what was being put forward. 'Angus swears nothing happened. He said he was in the lounge room with Sam and Olivia came in, yelling at him, then smacked his bottom really hard. He was so confused. I don't believe it's guilt he's feeling – it's just confusion. I should have screamed at her for hitting my child, but I just froze. I'm still scared of David myself. It's so stupid of me.'

The following day David called me. He told me to take Angus to a psychologist. He sounded like his old vile self. I tried my best to stay calm.

'He's acting out on Sam. I won't have it, Jack. He needs help. Liv won't have him back.' He hung up.

Finally, we agreed on something. I called Martyn and made an emergency appointment. Martyn's speciality was paediatric psychiatry, even though he'd see me over the age of forty. I took Angus with me and after a good chat with him he put us in contact with a paediatric psychologist who could fit us in within the week. Her name was Helen.

The first part of the appointment involved me speaking with Helen alone to explain what had happened. Angus then joined us and gave his interpretation of events. She asked him general questions about his personality but then she requested to see him the following week.

David still insisted that Olivia wasn't happy. I explained that Helen would be requesting both of them to visit her to work out what happened. I used the wrong terminology.

'I told you what fucking happened. I don't need to explain myself. He needs a good smack again.'

Then it rose up in me, something I should have said days earlier. 'David, if you want to see Angus again, you and Olivia will meet Helen. If you or your girlfriend lay a hand on our child, I will have you reported to the police. Do you understand?'

That started it.

Now he was yelling down the line. 'He's my child and I will not let him ruin my new family. You've gone and spoilt him. It's all your fault. He's a shark, Jack. He's a lying, little fucking shark. Angus can sense blood in the water, and if he thinks he's going to attack my newborn he's got another thing coming.' He sounded possessed.

'David, that's a crazy comment about Angus. You don't mean that.' Then I remembered what my old psychologist said to me to get David into her office.

Dr Lisa told me to always make it sound like I needed him to make everything better. 'Let him think he's in charge – make it about him.'

I lowered and calmed my voice, almost sounding desperate. The things I could do to change the game plan if it wasn't working, well, amazed me.

'David, we really need your input. We don't know what's wrong and we think you can help.'

His ego and pride snapped into place immediately. He took in a deep breath then exhaled loudly. 'OK.' He sounded like he was doing me a favour. 'I'll help you. I'm not sure if Liv will come but I'll ask. He needs help.' He now sounded like a spoilt child.

He made me sick. It wasn't making sense. The last thing I needed was David to take his anger out on Angus. Both medical professionals, Martyn and Helen, had spoken with Angus and they weren't picking up on any 'shark sensing blood' theory.

The following week David and Olivia made their way to meet and chat with Helen. The day after, I went in again with Angus. This happened for three weeks straight until David refused to return. He told me he wanted Angus to return to his house for a weekend. On a Thursday night, David called. 'I'll pick him up Friday night and drop him back to school Monday morning. Olivia has said he can come back into the house. Any trouble and you'll hear from me.' He was threatening me. He hung up.

I told Angus and thought he'd be happy that he could go back to see baby Sam again. He vomited on Friday morning.

'It's OK, sweetie. Don't be nervous. It'll be OK.'

'What happens if she hits me again?' He was so wide-eyed and scared.

I called David and told him Angus was sick; I couldn't let him go somewhere he didn't feel safe.

We were talking the following day though and Angus changed his mind, saying he wanted to go back to David's to see Sam.

'I do, Mum. I love Sam. I want to go.'

'I have an idea. Why don't you take Bear with you?'

Bear was a soft toy he'd been given when a friend of mine returned from Disneyland in Florida. Bear once had a clear Perspex space helmet on him but over time Angus had removed it so he could kiss him properly at night. Now Bear just had the Kennedy Space Centre logo needle pointed onto his chest, but it was truly cherished.

Angus declined to take Bear.

When Wednesday came around, Angus seemed to be better. I texted David that he was to pick Angus up after school.

As I was pulling our car into the kiss and drop point, I turned towards Angus. 'Give us a kiss and have a great time. Also why didn't you want to take Bear with you to Dad's?'

'I don't want Olivia to take him away too.'

'What do you mean?'

'She took all my toys away from my room. I don't have any toys now, so I don't want her to take Bear. 'Love you Mum. See ya.' With that, he kissed me and jumped out of the car to walk with his little friends to his classroom.

This was very wrong.

I made contact again with Helen, letting her know what Angus had told me. The most important part of this was to document everything that was going on so I started a paper diary. I only had an inside view to my son's life from his direct perspective or David's interpretation.

I was no longer in contact with David's mother or my sister-in-law Melissa. I'd been very close to both women. Ironically, it was these two women whom I missed more than anything when David and I broke up. I was dying to call them but I dared not in case David found out.

I also made extra appointments to see Martyn. I'd heard too many horror stories and seen too many examples of children being pulled apart by parents making bizarre accusations about the other's behaviour that ultimately left the children scared. I needed to see him to keep myself level headed about what I felt was going on around me or I wouldn't have ever been a help to Angus.

Then, after weeks of Angus being unsettled and David counteracting his words of worry, he was again at David's without a care. It was not unlike a child falling over, getting hurt and crying, then acting fine and wanting to go back on the playground. I was so worried and fearful about what had taken place, but then it was calm, as though I had nothing to worry about.

'Is everything at your Dad's, Angus?'

'Yep, it's good, Mum.'

'Really? Are you sure?'

'Mum, it's OK. It's fine.' He looked at me like I was interfering in his life.

'OK, but you let me know if you're not happy, OK?'

'Yep.'

It was constantly in the back of my mind that something was wrong and it wasn't going to settle then go away. It took weeks for me to feel safe with the decision to allow Angus to be with his dad's new family. Apart from work and my art, I needed another outlet; I was overthinking everything way too much.

I'd signed on to an online dating site a few months previous. I'd filled out the pages of questions like I was doing a Myers Briggs personality indicator test, and then closed my laptop. I poured a glass of Sav B because I was mentally exhausted and forgot about it. Out of the blue, months later I received an email via the platform from a man called Jason. He'd been sent to me as a match a week prior but I'd just ignored it as so much had been going on. He wanted to know if he could email me. Oddly enough, he happened to be an ex-work colleague of an old friend of mine from high school. Jason's email was very kind, but then I thought that of so many others that came before him. I decided to accept his correspondence. I told him that I wasn't looking for anything other than just friends to start with and he replied in the positive. We emailed back and forth for a few weeks, then we texted and eventually spoke on the phone.

Our words to one another were just typical banter about nothing in particular. He opened up about his life and told me he had a daughter who was fifteen. He'd split with his wife eighteen months prior but there was no animosity in his words – they were just getting on with their lives separately and raising their daughter respectively. Her name was Darcy.

I'd found a new email friend. With everything else that had been going on, it was nice to sit down and get my day out in a letter of sorts. I never spoke ill of anyone around me though – it wasn't anyone else's business. Jason was very polite and we spoke about anything and everything, but not at all romance-based. It never went into a sexual territory; it was just like chatting with an old friend, one who was witty and very intelligent. We formed a good friendship.

Eventually, one night the topic arrived at health and it was then that I decided to tell Jason about being bipolar. I would never have shared that information previously to strangers as people always looked too straight-faced then would almost back away. It was quite comical to watch even though I didn't find it funny.

Jason happened to mention a drug his doctor had put him on for epilepsy. I thought, *I'm going to tell him the truth and if it freaks him out so be it.* But it didn't. He kept chatting like I'd just told him I took a Panadol for a headache.

'Jason, do you know what bipolar is? Bipolar 2, to be exact.'
'Yeah, I think.'
'OK, if you don't understand it, I can't explain it, if you want.'
'OK.'

It was that simple. I explained the major points of living with a serious mental illness. I wanted him to understand that it was something that I controlled with drugs but I'd never be cured of it. He never judged me. He knew what it meant – the highs, the lows, the lot. When we spoke again after that night, he asked me on a date. We were to meet for the first time, just after a month of chatting. We were going to meet for lunch in Carlton.

It was a beautiful Melbourne day in late August and spring had decided to pop in early. I was sitting in my car on Alexandra Parade in bumper-to-bumper traffic and I had my finger on speed dial. I was close to cancelling. I'd driven the whole way into the city to meet Jason for the first time and all I could hear was my hairdresser's voice in my head, telling me horror stories for the two hours it took for a regrowth, a couple of highlights and a blow wave. Dreaded tails of hook-up bankruptcy for the whole visit. I walked out of that appointment with so many horror stories about men doing terrible things to women I was shocked and that's saying something for someone who advocates for abused women. So, no one could have blamed me for actually calling Jason and saying, 'Thanks but no thanks'.

And there were those signs I was looking for again. I was praying I couldn't find a park on the busy road so I could call and tell him that it was the reason we couldn't meet. Bugger – I found a car park right near the restaurant. I tried to compose myself. I took a deep breath, convinced that I was about to make the biggest mistake. He was a lovely guy but I was a repeat offender in finding dickheads.

As I walked, I caught the first rays of sun on my face after winter. It was warm and so beautiful. There Jason was, sitting outside the restaurant on busy Lygon Street. As I walked up to him to introduce myself, I put out my hand. He stood, shaking it. It was as though I was hit with an electrical jolt, and no, I wasn't walking on synthetic carpet before you think it was static electricity I felt.

It sounds so bloody cheesy and romantic – and I don't do romantic cheesy – but this was an instant connection. In all my years I'd never felt it.

We took a seat inside, facing the street, and we chatted for four hours. It was so comfortable. His voice was deep but calming. He was intelligent but not a tosser. He was polite and it wasn't awkward. It was a lovely afternoon – so easy.

A second lunch date followed the next Saturday, at the same restaurant. We happened to, funnily enough, buy each other a small gift. It was so random that we both bought each other fridge magnets. Jason's said something beautiful like: *Every goal that has ever been reached began with just one step. And the belief that it could be attained. Believe in yourself and remember that I believe in you, too. By J. Blume.*

Mine to him had a woman with a glass of whiskey in her hand and read: *E-Harmony Matched Me with Jack Daniels.*

He walked me to my car and we kissed goodbye. It was so natural. I really liked this person – a lot.

The panic hit more so when I got home and, as it surged through me, I realised what I feared the most. What I felt with Jason was a strong emotional pull; I didn't trust something that was so based on emotions. It never worked, like ever. I was pacing my bathroom, staring at myself in the mirror and talking to myself – like it was really logical. I didn't want passion, I didn't want exciting, I didn't want to be impulsive. I felt nervous around this man, but it wasn't a feeling of grievance, it was butterflies and I didn't want them. I didn't want to feel skittish. Skittish was romance-based and I didn't want to be anywhere near that. No, no, no. I wanted to be in control. Being in control was soothing, knowing I had discipline in my relationships was calming; but this wasn't it. I needed to call the shots because then I'd feel safe, but that wasn't happening.

Seeing my car in the carport after the second date, Jane popped over with my spare key in her hand and heard me talking to someone. She caught me in the act of holding a full-on dialogue with myself.

'What are you going on about? You sound crazy—Oh, hang on, you are.' She started laughing at her own original joke.

'Yeah, you're hilarious. What am I going to do? This is really bad.'

I was so upset. It was too much to feel for something that I wanted to be slow and steady. 'What if he's a complete and utter tosser like the others I've had a brilliant track record with?'

'I get it. You don't trust yourself, and you don't trust anyone else currently. I can't change the situation – only you can do that. What I can do is ask you to breathe and know that I may have done something slightly immoral, especially since it entailed a good friend of mine and her job in detention centres. But I only did it for a) Angus, b) because I love you and c) you have, as you say, a terrible track record. Wanna know what it is?' She looked sneaky, raising her eyebrows and smiling.

I nodded.

'Well, I asked Sonia to run a check on Jason, and guess what? She didn't find a record for him, so isn't that great?'

'YOU WHAT?'

'It's not illegal. It might be morally wrong but, as you say, you never know what's lurking out there these days. Let's be honest, you haven't been with a lot of men but the ones you've been with have been complete and utter psychopaths, except Charlie, and that was your choice, so I'm trying to limit the grief.'

She wasn't being overly dramatic either. I wasn't a good judge of character.

She continued. 'Jason sounds almost too good, to be honest, Jack. But I haven't got any connections with the Victorian Police or ASIO so it'll have to do.' She looked proud.

It was at that time that I had to decide whether to pivot from the fear of my past choices and choose to start a serious relationship or drop what was in front of me. It had to be weighed up before I took the next step, but to weigh up my options involved thinking about the most important person in all of this: Angus.

It was something I discussed with Jason. I let him know my feelings that Angus would always be the number one priority in my life, no questions asked. It was what he expected as well, as Darcy would be his priority too.

It's my belief that when a pyramid of care breaks down, where a partner or parent puts the other first before their child, it opens up an opportunity for abuse and exploitation to occur. A child needs to know they are safe no matter what external events may happen through their life. I didn't have that as a child but Angus would.

From two people who started off slowly chatting via email and then on the phone, we decided to give the relationship a shot. We were opposites in many ways but so complementary in others. Jason was lateral thinking, logical and composed. My work was based on being creative, but he did his best work on a spreadsheet. We are an example of how two extremes can coincide and still be equal. I'd not had such balance in a relationship before, even with Charlie, because I gave my power away. I felt I needed men to 'take charge'. When they didn't, I was lost.

It's a good feeling knowing you and your child are safe and understanding that there's no hidden agenda. No one was lying or going behind my back. Everything was equal. It was official: I had started dating a feminist. There's strength in knowing your partner is behind you one hundred percent. Whatever choice you make they will say, 'Go for it. If it doesn't work, it's no big deal'. My internal reply would normally have been, 'What's the catch?' There wasn't one.

I had my red flag senses out from day one, as did Jane and Andrew, but he was true to his word. His only requests in life were as follows:

- He doesn't do handyman jobs around the house, as he doesn't want to put a tradie out of a job. (Funnily enough, we do flat packs really well together.)

- He says all he needs is a cosy couch to relax on each night.

- That Foxtel be available for his large flat screen TV to watch AFL in winter and cricket in summer.

- A comfortable bed to sleep in at the end of the day.

It was that simple, or so I thought. After two months of being in a 'love bubble', things became very contorted. At first it showed itself as I was going about my day, reflecting on what I'd entered into and then it would appear as this dark obscurity that I wasn't deserving of someone who was decent. Or was he decent? I couldn't give away complete control as I'd done in the past. He insisted on paying for bills that I'd handled before. I understood that, because he was spending so much time at my place, he was only being considerate. Him paying for any of the utilities would scare me so much I started to hide them from him, then delay paying them all together. It was such erratic behaviour on my part. Bills have a due date and I knew they needed to be paid. Because he told me to pay them, I held off – I wasn't doing what he expected, what he wanted, what was normal behaviour. Again, I needed to be in control, but not paying bills isn't logical. I'd receive overdue notices, even though I had the money to handle my bills. It was crazy.

My paranoia kicked in and I came up with some of the most elaborate plans that he was going to do something unthinkable to majorly screw me over. Honestly, if my thoughts had played out onto the pages of a psychological thriller, I could have made a lot of money. Patricia Cornwell would've been very impressed.

Then it bled into the bedroom. What started out as a beautiful connection between two people expressing their love for one another became a battle in my mind. I wanted sex to be rough. I wanted to hurt and be hurt, treated as though I wasn't worthy of anything so special. Jason was showing his commitment to me and all I had was an overwhelming sense that I wanted to be hit. I wanted to be struck so I'd bleed. He wouldn't do it though. At times I was so angry, he'd pull away horrified, standing up out of bed.

'Don't, Jack. I can't do it. You don't understand how strong I can be. I just can't do it.' He'd look so deflated, defeated.

Let me put this into perspective weight wise too: Jason was over 100 kilograms and built like a rugby union player. I, on the other hand, was weighing in the featherweight division, at best 57 kilograms.

When I didn't get my way, which was always, I'd get up and have a shower to scrub myself, feeling so much anger that he wouldn't meet my demand. So simple – just abuse me.

Each time in the end he just held me. He'd wrap his huge arms around my naked body, his legs intertwined in mine and speak to soothe me. He would try and stop the ominous agitation. I'd attempt to pull away again but he'd keep holding me gently, talking softly until I gave up. He'd pull the doona over me, my medication finally pulling me into a deep sleep. He never wavered though – he had the conviction to lie by my side each night and calm me until it stopped. He wasn't going anywhere.

In the background was my counsellor Sophie. For weeks on end she would talk not only to me, but to Jason as well, helping me to recalibrate my idea of what a healthy relationship was (or wasn't, more to the point). Red flags were ablaze, showing themselves in glorious full colour but only for my behaviour, no one else's. It was time to be responsible, to accept what was in front of me. It was time to learn to breathe through the agitation and simply welcome the love that was on offer.

I had reached another point, another hurdle where I decided I would at least try. Trying didn't mean it would be easy. Each day seemed to bring a challenge and I had to push through it. I was slowly learning that I could accomplish the simplest of things that before were unachievable. If I screwed up, then I had to try again if I felt it was worth it. I was now one half of a team and the other half was trying so hard to understand my behaviour when sometimes I couldn't even verbalise it. Jason never gave up; he doesn't give up on anything he wants or, more importantly, on anyone he loves.

I accepted that I'd met my best friend. Someone who made me laugh and who was there for both Angus and I no matter what. There was no underlying reason, there was no glorious performance hidden behind an agenda. It was simply this: I'd met a person who accepted me for who I was. He loved both Angus and I without exception. My whole family could see that he adored us and all he wanted was for us to be happy and secure in our new life together.

From the beginning I was very open about my challenges, but didn't go into all the specific details. I needed to test the waters to see if he'd run away. He didn't, but it wasn't easy for him, as Jason will explain.

'I grew up with a father who hit my mother; therefore to me if a man beats a woman, it is one of the lowest acts a man can ever perform.

'I couldn't understand why Jack didn't have boundaries. I said I was fine with a little rough foreplay but when I saw she wanted much more it scared me. It could have been truly harmful. I could see in full view that she had lost respect for herself.'

The more intimate our love became, the more he wanted me to learn to love again and let someone love me properly. He knew that was going to take time.

'It was during this same period that I saw other traits that she struggled with; her past would vividly pop back into her head and she'd land back in bed, curled up and sobbing. To be left alone in the dark was all she wanted, and it was horrible to see as all I wanted was to fix it and I couldn't.

'I'd become so angry. I didn't handle the situation well at all, which would lead us to fighting, screaming at each other, which would get her even more upset. It was never my intention though. I simply didn't know what I was dealing with. But, instead of walking out, over time I became better at looking for the signs of what would be her triggers and the occurrences become less frequent.

'When things were calm, it was wonderful. We are so in love. What I couldn't understand was we were happy. Our lifestyle was pretty comfortable, better than the last couple of years with her struggling as a single parent, much better than the years with David. We travelled, ate out, we could afford for Angus to do fun activities with his mates that she couldn't afford before – life was good. What I didn't realise was that it was an absolute battle in her mind.'

Unfortunately, all I could think of was, *Why is this man being so nice to me?* It was so foreign. What had I done to deserve his kindness? I couldn't accept my new life; it was so normal but ultimately that's what made it wrong. Jason kept reminding me that the past may have shaped me as a person but it didn't define me anymore so, again, I had a choice to make. It was then I took a deep breath and stepped into my new life –a healthier one.

2016 – September

For all its challenges, life at home was good, but it didn't last long. David was getting more upset about Angus. When he came to pick him up for outings, he started to berate him before he got in the car about how he needed to behave around Olivia or he wouldn't be allowed to come over as often. I wanted to stop him from going to his dad's but he still insisted until a night in September when Angus was invited to a birthday party for one of his friends.

Angus was never a shy child and enjoyed his friends' company, but that night he wasn't himself. He stared crying each time someone accidentally knocked him when they were playing games. As the party grew to a close, he started to become so scared that I called David to tell him he wasn't well and wouldn't be coming over. He wasn't having any of it and started yelling at me that he expected Angus to be delivered to him. I told David I had to get Angus to the doctors. I resorted to lying to keep him away from Angus, but it wasn't going to keep him away for good.

The following weekend Angus said he wanted to go again, saying he missed his dad, Sam and Anouk. It became this perpetual stopping and starting of not wanting to go to David's and then changing his mind. I still stayed in contact with the paediatric psychologist, Helen, as I didn't know how to deal with the normal fluctuating moods of a child. I was trying to balance a child in two minds and an ex-husband trying to throw his weight around. It was about to get worse.

Jason and I had only started to become serious in our relationship and, even though he had met Angus and I had met his daughter Darcy, the kids were yet to meet one another.

David and Olivia had recently become engaged. In the beginning of November they were planning to get married. When I questioned Angus if he was happy for his dad, he said he didn't care.

Whenever David dropped Angus off, he refused to come to the front door. He knew Jason was inside and he didn't want to have direct contact with him. It was obvious that he was offended there was another man in my life. One afternoon, I met Angus outside when David dropped him home. Angus went to give me a hug. David started telling me that he was extremely disappointed with Angus' behaviour of late. He and Olivia had decided not to have him as a part of their wedding.

'What? Not be a pageboy? That's a bit harsh.'

'No. Not attending at all.'

Surely I'd misheard. I had a hopeful smile on my face as though I was at fault for my lack of hearing. I wasn't.

'Liv and I are serious about this. It's our special day and we don't want him ruining it,' he said, staring down at our son.

Angus already knew the drill and looked blasé towards David's changed plan. I thought he'd be more upset.

'Angus, did you know about this?' I asked.

'Yeah. Dad and Livy told me they didn't want me to ruin their day.'

Typical kid – he just spoke the truth. He could have of easily said, 'Dad wants me to take out the rubbish bin'. It was that casual.

I looked into David's eyes. 'Does Granny Emmie know? This isn't right, David. You're getting married and he should be there. You can't exclude him. He's your child.' I'm sure I almost sounded like I was pleading. I just couldn't believe it. 'Angus, say goodbye to your dad please and go inside.'

Angus hugged David and left. I asked him about Granny Emmie again.

Granny Emmie and Angus were inseparable. They had an incredible bond from the time he was born and I was sure she'd have something to say even if I hadn't seen her for years.

'I don't give a shit what she thinks. It's none of her fucking business. And don't call her.' He was now pointing his finger towards my chest, just like the old days, but this time he knew he couldn't physically touch me.

Red flag: his relationship with his mother was getting worse.

'Why are you being so cruel to him? I don't understand.'

'Do you remember a few weeks ago when we took Angus with us to a family wedding, and do you know what he did?' He kept on talking over me. 'Angus cried like a baby. He was an embarrassment to the family. He's so weak.'

Red flag: the spite in his tone was apparent when talking about his own child.

'David, that wedding was on a Friday night straight after school and I know you didn't give him anything to eat before he went. It was a double ceremony that took three hours, you told me so. What time did he eat?'

'It was an Indian ceremony and there was an enormous amount of food.'

'OK, let's do the math.'

'Jackie, you can't count so that's not going to happen.'

He was right. I wasn't gifted with a mathematical brain but I gave it a good shot.

I put my index finger up in protest. 'Bear with me, it's only simple math. You collected him from school a few hours after he ate lunch, then drove twenty-five minutes back to your place to get him and you dressed, minimum forty-five minutes to get back in the car to leave.'

He went to speak. Now it was my time to speak over him, and I was pissed off. 'Stop interrupting! I was married to you, spent six, unfortunately unforgettable years with you. I should know! You drove to the other side of the city on a Friday afternoon. That can take at least an hour and a half. Then sat through a three-hour ceremony. That's at least seven and a half hours without anything, not even a snack. I know your pattern. You think of no one but yourself and your behaviour towards our son is disgusting.'

He raised his finger at me again, but I turned before he could speak, then turned back at a safe distance.

'And stop pointing at me. You'll accidently poke a hole in the sky.'

Seriously the stuff that came out of my mouth when I was pushed to a point astounded me!

I quickly walked back into the house. I felt sick at his lack of regard for his own child. I went straight to Angus' room.

'Are you OK? He's not here now. He can't hurt you. Tell me what happened.'

'At the wedding Granny Emmie took me to the food to eat while those people were getting married and Daddy got angry with me. Then he had a big fight with Granny.'

Red flag: Granny Emmie is on the outer again.

'What did he say about you not going to his wedding to Olivia?'

'She told Anouk and I to sit at the table as a lady was coming over to organise the ceremony. She said if the lady asks me if I'm going to the wedding I had to say no. I wasn't going to be invited.'

Red flag: Olivia is excluding Angus from everything to do with the family.

'What did Dad say?'

'She told him and then he agreed with her.'

Red flag: they were both excluding him.

Again I asked Angus if he wanted to skip going to David's the following second weekend, but he insisted he go. I kept him at home for the overnight stays in between and he said he missed Anouk. 'She's kind to me Mum and I want to see Sam.' He was collected by David that Friday.

The following day, I was in the passenger seat driving with Jason to collect Darcy from her mother's. Not long after leaving my home, I received a frantic call from David, telling me I had to come over immediately as Angus had attacked Olivia. I couldn't believe what I was hearing. It didn't make sense. Had Angus just snapped with Olivia? Was he pushed? I was in shock but I was looking for a rational reason. Immediately Jason changed direction and headed to David's. As I walked up, the door opened. Angus was standing there. The clothes he was in looked dishevelled and didn't fit him properly – his ankles were bare and his jumper had holes in it. He'd been crying. All David could tell me was that Olivia had put Angus in his room for being naughty, then when she went to get him out of his room, he hit her.

'Angus, did you hit Olivia?'

He nodded. 'Yes.'

I wanted to hear exactly what happened away from David. I didn't want his bullying tactics invading Angus' mind and twisting his words. If his behaviour was bad, I needed to deal with it alone. He had never behaved in that way, ever. I took Angus' hand and got him into the car. Jason drove us back to his house in silence. I went blank; the drive takes an hour but I lost track of time in my own mind again. I needed to process what happened. I couldn't speak and I didn't want to hear anything. I zoned out, praying that the truth would come out. David lied continually but Angus had just admitted to hitting Olivia. What the hell was going on? Jason could see my distress and took my hand as he drove through the rain. All I focused on to keep from losing control was each tiny roll of reflective silver water rolling down the car window's exterior.

I wanted to roll up into the smallest ball and disappear. I didn't want to be present but that would mean ignoring the truth and I'd watched my mother do that brilliantly. That wasn't an option. I knew better, no matter how disturbing it was. I had to stand up and face it head on but with a level head.

'Just breathe. It'll be OK. We'll work it out.' Jason was so kind but it was my problem, not his.

We were inside the apartment and we sat Angus down to watch some TV. I was in another room, trying to process something I had no idea how I was going to tackle. All I could think was what had I done? What had I done to allow this event to occur? That's how I process major events, and from the outside it can look as though I've frozen. It's the fear of choosing what is the truth and what isn't. I had to go to my son, this eight-year-old child, and hear his story as to what happened through his eyes. I wasn't my mother; I wanted to know my son's truth. It was Angus who I needed to hear; he knew I didn't tolerate lying. He needed to tell me what went on. I knew but I feared I wouldn't know how to resolve it.

I wiped away my tears and went to where Angus was sitting. I gently turned off the television and knelt down so we were looking directly at each other.

'What happened, Gus? Just tell me the truth from the very start.'

He started slowly, looking shy. 'She sent me to my room again. She made me say to my dad that I was sick, but I wasn't sick. I have to stay in my bedroom or they send me to Granny Emmie's to stay. I like that better. She told me I couldn't come out of my bedroom or she'd get really mad with me. She told me she didn't want to see me.' He continued. 'Each weekend she said it, but this weekend I said no, and then I hit her. Anouk walked in and said, "Did you hit my mum?" I told her yes.' He was nodding his head, agreeing with the statement he'd made. Now he was crying.

I held him gently. 'Go on, I'm listening.'

'Livy said yes too. They put me in the cold hall way … '

There was a back hallway in David's house and it was almost glacial, any time of the year. Nothing could warm it. It didn't have any windows and it was on the low side of a block of land that was extremely damp. It was dank.

'I was there for a long time and Anouk came in and made fun of me and I kicked her. Then Livy came back in and Anouk told her, then she kicked me.'

'Olivia kicked you?'

He nodded. 'Dad heard what I did when he woke up and she told him. And then he called you.' He continued. 'I hated her before Sam came. She's been mean to me for a long time. I don't want to see her again.'

'Don't worry, you won't. You won't go back ever again.'

'But I want to see Daddy.' He was looking at me scared. 'I'm sorry. I don't want Daddy to be angry with me. I want to see Daddy.'

Now tears were rolling again down my face as I held him close. I had my little boy in my arms, crying because he was scared, needing his father's love and approval and completely confused as to why he wasn't adored by either of the adults meant to protect him.

'I just want to go back and say I'm sorry. I won't do it again. I wanna go back.'

'Angus, I know you won't understand this but you won't be going back there for a while.'

In my mind I knew it wouldn't be for a long time but in my heart I felt it would be forever. I couldn't let my child go back into a toxic environment where he wasn't loved and cared for.

'I want Dad.' He was crying and it was the most heartbreaking thing to ever go through.

Jason then came back into the room and sat with us. 'Angus, would you like to watch a movie? This was one of Darcy's favourite when she was little.'

He peeked his head around to see what Jason was putting on Foxtel.

'She's so looking forward to meeting you. I've just spoken with her; would you like to meet her?'

He nodded shyly. He was always happy to meet new people.

It broke my heart that the person he loved more than anything didn't want to love him back. And my strong feelings of always making it a priority that this father and son should have the best possible relationship possible didn't matter. It was another example of delusional happiness, something that wasn't going to exist. If it were it would be only on David's terms and I wouldn't let my son live in a relationship based on pleasing others as I had done in the past.

It wasn't unlike the relationship I'd had with my father. Just because you put yourself out there expecting your parent to love you as you do them, it doesn't guarantee adoration in return. Sometimes even for a parent to simply like you isn't achievable.

I'd made a decision then that he wouldn't return to David's home as I'd wished my mother had protected me from my father. I used to pray as a small child that Mum would leave Dad, that we could go away and be happy. I bore a child and it was automatic that I felt this love for him as I'd never loved another. It was all-powerful, pure and unbreakable. Through anything I will love him but his father obviously never had it. I thought he did but that was to be another illusion I conjured up or that I thought true.

David would often use the words 'my boy'. This absolute statement that he owned Angus, but he was never 'ours'. He's his own little person and we were blessed that he chose us as parents. The day I found out I was pregnant I knew a) it was a boy and b) he was going to teach me so much. Oddly enough I never wanted a girl, back then I felt I had been too much trouble to deal with, and I couldn't go through it; my thought was that boys had a better shot at life. This was one hell of a lesson. I knew that he was always my number one priority. That was instinctive. I had this fine line to balance between keeping a little boy happy and safe. I grappled with going to the police and yet I didn't – it's something I still battle with. I had to sit with being uncomfortable and think then act, knowing I'd chosen the best outcome. I couldn't allow myself to react. I'd done a lot of reacting in my past life and it had never worked out well for me and I wasn't about to throw Angus into the depth of a drama. It was already bad enough.

I wrote everything down, then deliberated.

- Angus was eight.

- David had not protected him, and had stood by his fiancée instead.

- Angus admitted hitting then kicking Olivia.

- David was threatening to never see his son again.

I had a little boy who was so in love with his father. He looked up to him, and to steal that away would devastate Angus. All he said he wanted was to see his father. I needed to find a solution without disagreement or retribution from anyone, and I even asked him.

'Angus, this is very serious what Olivia did to you. She's a grown-up and should have known better. She shouldn't have touched you or treated you that way. We can go to the police.'

'No, Mum. I don't want that.'

Very simple instructions. I didn't want to take him to the police station and have him deny everything because he was scared.

Angus had grown up in a household with a mother who had been so ill that, at times, things had been disjointed for him. I needed to find something that would give him stability and normality in his world. Something so simple: love. I just wanted him to be loved by both parents, no matter what we felt towards each other. I thought it wasn't a lot to ask for. I was obviously wrong.

2016 – November

I'd made my decision. I couldn't let Angus suffer any longer for David's pitiful mistake of not looking after his son and leaving him with a woman who obviously hated him. We decided that there was only to be visitation rights, with David coming to our place to collect him for four hours per week on a Sunday afternoon.

When Angus returned one afternoon he was happy. David had taken him for a milkshake and they played basketball alone together. No interference from anyone. The rhythm of the two of them meeting like that went on for a month until one afternoon David broached a request.

'I need to ask a favour.' He was straight-faced this time.

'Oh, you've reminded me, I need to ask you a favour first. I don't know what you've done with Gus' clothes. Every time that I've sent him to your place they're never returned with him. Can I please have them back? I'm not made of money,' I said.

'Sure, whatever.'

'I'm serious. When he stayed with you, you were sending him home in worn-out jocks. I make sure he has new underwear constantly but for some reason they aren't coming back and I'm ending up with a draw full of holey underwear that I didn't buy. Angus said they are from Olivia's nephew Noah. Is that true? Were you putting him in second-hand jocks?'

He looked at me blankly, shrugging his shoulders. 'I have no idea, I'll check.'

He knew damn well what was going on but again lied. He lived in a house well over a million dollars and our son was in holey second-hand underwear. His and Olivia's frugal behaviour was damning. He was so irritating.

'What do you want anyway? You said you wanted a favour. Please entertain me. What could you possibly want me to do … for you?'

'I'm getting married this Friday night and I'd like to see Angus.'

'What? At the wedding?' There it was again: my astonishment at his requests.

'No, not the wedding service. I'd like to see him before the wedding. I was hoping I could pick him up after school on Friday around 2 pm and then drop him back to you around 4 pm at your work? Please, I need to see him before I go away.'

I straightened up. My speech became clearer so he could understand what I was saying. 'David, do you realise how pathetic that request is? Many people see you as an intelligent man, I have no idea why, but do you not hear how insane you sound having settled on the decision not to let Angus attend your own wedding?'

He took a deep breath, and sounded almost worn out. 'Please.'

I turned to Angus, simplifying hid dad's request. 'Do you want to?'

'Yes, Mum.'

'David, you're lucky this time I asked him. Next time I won't even bother, so don't ask.'

As said, he collected Angus from school on the Friday and dropped him off to me at work at 4 pm. It was a beautiful afternoon and as soon as Angus was returned, he said his goodbyes to his dad and left to go and sit in my office. It was then I had a strong feeling that it was good that Angus had had time with his dad to make memories for the future. It was an odd feeling; it was like he wouldn't see him again. It was over. I turned and walked away as he drove out into the busy Friday evening traffic.

The following Wednesday was basketball night for Angus' school's team. The smell of the stadium always hit me; it's the same as the sound. The aromatic reminiscence of smelly socks and body odour matched with interrupted pounding of sneakers on polished wooden boards and the occasional squeak of rubber as a foot changed direction due to an official whistle being blown.

Angus smiled and headed over to meet his mates as I tried to find the most comfortable position one can find on a hard-wooden bench. I was four benches high so I had a good spot to see everything. Surprisingly, a local unknown number popped up on my phone. I answered.

'Good afternoon. It's Sonia calling from the Child Support Agency. Am I speaking with Jacqueline Ellwood?'

I rolled my eyes; I knew the drill by now. They called me, I answered with my name, they'd get me to repeat what we both already knew, including my date of birth and the mobile number they'd called me on. Genius.

'Can I please also confirm that you are the mother to Angus Fredrick Billings?'

'I am.' I smiled but also breathed out a big sigh. I didn't mean to be rude; Sonia was obviously only doing her job. But I'd just driven through peak school traffic. I was half-frazzled knowing I had to get home and have dinner on the table pretty quickly as Angus would be starving. His appetite matched his height; both were getting bigger.

'Jacqueline, I'm calling you to advise you of a change of care. Angus' father, David Billings, has formally requested that you now will have one hundred percent care of Angus as of today.'

Sonia read me the date. I went blank. Rejection was flooding me. But not for me, for Angus. It stung terribly. Time stopped.

'Jacqueline, are you there?' Sonia asked.

'Ah, yes, yes, I'm here. What do I do now?' I still didn't understand completely what she was saying – or just couldn't believe it – and now I needed to wake up and get further information to help this next drama stabilise before I told Angus. It wasn't unlike running around trying to catch burning embers with my bare hands. I was astounded.

'Nothing for now, we've posted you a letter of confirmation and David's monthly payments to Angus will remain the same. Is there anything else we can help you with today?'

Did they help me though? Was it a help knowing that David had decided not to have any caring rights for his son?

I stood in the corner of court three in a suburban basketball stadium watching Angus play with his little friends. He was none the wiser. His father had just relinquished any care of him. I hung my head in disbelief. The game ended and I walked towards Angus. He was 'too old' to have his hand held; I wasn't though. We walked to the car.

'Great game, Gus,' I told him on our way home.

My day should have been winding down then, but I was just getting started.

2016 – November

Two days after I received the call from Child Support, I finally received confirmation in the mail. My heart broke for my son. This decision David made was incorrect. It was a mistake, inappropriate, just wrong. Terribly wrong. Heartbreak was eventually interrupted with vile anger. I decided to take it out on someone close to David, as I couldn't get hold of him. I dialled my ex-mother-in-law, Granny Emmie. It rang. She picked up.

'Emelia, it's Jackie. David's ex-wife.'

I had a speech planned but she frantically interrupted.

'Oh my God. I've been trying to call you, Jackie, but I didn't have your number. I must have lost it. I was thinking of going to Scarlett's parents' house to get Scarlett to give you a message. Where was Angus? He wasn't at the wedding.'

Granny Emmie lived near Scarlett's parents and, as she didn't drive, she had no other way of contacting me.

It was typical that David had left everyone in the dark about Angus not being at his nuptials. I wanted Emmie to pay for her son's incompetence towards our child. I wanted her to know that I was going to hunt David down when he returned to Melbourne and make him pay for what he and his new wife had done to Angus. I could barely convey what I felt and then she allowed an insight from her perspective.

'Jackie, I haven't seen Angus for months. I'm going crazy. He was meant to be at the wedding and he wasn't there. Why I don't know? I kept asking where he was and David wouldn't say anything. He's a pig, and I need to see my baby boy. Can I see him? When can you bring him to me?' She was panicked.

David had shafted his mother too. And so, the next hour was spent filling each other in on the goings-on over the few years that we hadn't seen each other. We were joining the dots as to what each other knew. It was like piecing together a puzzle of happenings that I wasn't privy to. I heard about things that made my temper run even higher. She told me that just before Angus had attacked Olivia, he went missing one afternoon when David had dropped him off to Emmie's as Olivia didn't want him around their house any longer. They hunted for an hour over her house and land and were just about to call the police when they found him hiding in her pantry. He had curled himself into a ball, scared of being taken back to David's house. David pulled Angus out by the scruff of the jumper, smacked him hard and loaded him in his car. Emmie never saw him again.

There were stories of brand new clothes going missing that had been bought for Angus. She'd buy him clothes, even give him money in the hundreds, which would never be seen again, let alone by Angus himself. I'd always made sure Angus was well dressed for his family outings if he had to go out with David, but the clothes were never returned to me. It was more than I cared to think of.

She explained that she had disliked Olivia from the beginning. Something wasn't right with her and the whole family thought so. Olivia wasn't even kind to Anouk. Emmie said that Olivia and her had come to blows many times. David had told her to butt out and chosen a partner over his family as well as his own son.

When I finally got off the phone from her, promising to take him over the following weekend, I was exhausted. I crawled into bed but didn't sleep well. I still hadn't told Angus and I feared how he'd react. Jane and Anne had advised me not to tell him – they thought he was too young. Angus was at the centre of this debacle. I felt that I needed to explain to him the truth so he could at least acknowledge it but still feel the love that everyone felt for him. It wasn't his fault and he needed to be involved in the discussion. I needed to not make a big deal of it but we needed to deal with it as a family, just him and I.

I took him to a local park so we could chat and play at the same time.

'Angus, I need to tell you something and it involves your dad.'

I had to stay neutral. He looked at me waiting for me to talk again.

'I got a letter the other day from him and he's asked to have a break from seeing you for a while.'

'Is it because of Olivia?'

'Yes, I think so.'

'It's all her fault, and I don't want to go anyway.' He shrugged his shoulders

'That's OK,' I said.

'I want to see the letter.'

Bugger – I didn't want to show him but I'd taken it just in case. I passed the folded note to him.

'So, I'll never see Dad again.' We were swinging in unison on the play equipment.

'You know what, Gus? I feel you will but it won't be for a while. You'll be older when you see him again.' I'd always been truthful with him.

'Can I go on the slide now?'

'For sure. Can you promise me one thing though?'

He nodded.

'Any time you want to talk about this at home, I'm here. And do you know Mrs Williams at school? Well, I've told her so you can chat with her Monday morning and any time you want to.'

Mrs Williams was the school's counsellor.

Photocopies of the letter were distributed to the principal and his teachers. David was no longer allowed on the school's property to see Angus. If he tried I had it put in the file that the police were to be called. His school reports were to be no longer emailed to him. He had lost all privileges regarding Angus. He was now officially irrelevant to raising him. I refused to let his fatherly incompetence take a toll on either of us. We'd get through this together, no matter what.

It did take a toll on my relationship with Jason, though. I had this enormous feeling come over me for weeks to follow that I had to wipe the slate clean from anything that wasn't direct family. I felt I had to start anew – things would be perfect if I eradicated the past, including Jason.

Jason, as always, was incredibly stoic in a time where everything seemed to be sinking. It was at that time that he told me he was committed to raising Angus alongside me and that he considered him his son. And true to his word, from that day on he said he had two children, Darcy and Angus. My little boy adored that he now had a big sister who he loved unconditionally and a supportive and strong role model in his stepdad Jason. For me, I'd finally gotten the family I'd always wanted. We were now four and our home was always full of love. Love – something so simple. It isn't a lot to ask for, is it?

2015-2016

Dad was diagnosed with the early signs of dementia and one day in frustration Mum told him to go and do some gardening. He headed to the rose garden, which was on a slope and covered in large rocks. He took a tumble that resulted in him breaking his neck. After he was released from The Alfred hospital, he was bedridden in a neck brace for the next month in a rehab hospital. We all took it in turns visiting each day, but he was in no mind to be rehabilitated. From that point, he had given up trying.

Once Dad was back home, I took time off work to help Mum get him to doctor's appointments. He was admitted to hospital on many occasions as he was also suffering a heart murmur. On the fourth release I had to step in and tell the nursing staff that he couldn't be returned home as he was starting to physically threaten Mum with harm. We were both scared of his behaviour.

If you've ever been looking for a decent facility for your aged parents, you know the drill. Appointments were made and home after home was visited, only to be told there was a waiting list for any that didn't smell of urine and bleach. For those that didn't, it would cost a fortune.

Mum only had one request that I found unsettling: she wanted a home where he would be served a glass of wine with dinner. He barely knew his name, not to mention wanting to partake in his nightly drinking sessions. I'm sure she felt guilty. She was so concerned he'd be missing his Shiraz.

I couldn't quite work out why nobody ever spoke about what it's like when your parents reach a time in their lives where they need parenting. It was crazy. Maybe it was because I was the oldest of my girlfriends – they had yet to go into the void that it is. And don't even mention the paperwork involved. Again, it's pure bureaucracy, be it a state- or federal-run home.

We finally found somewhere close to Mum. She visited Dad every second day. When she to attempted to visit more often, he'd just verbally abuse her and it took its toll.

In the same week we got him settled, I drove her to a well overdue appointment with a surgical oncologist at Cabrini Hospital. I drove her home an hour later with a diagnosis of bowel cancer. She kept trying to make light of it but the oncologist insisted she be operated on within five days. The day of the operation I drove her in and sat with her until she was prepared for theatre and then wheeled into a waiting area to be retrieved by the nursing staff. They put a warmed blanket on her and I could see the fear in her face. I held her hand and we both cried, unsure of the outcome. She explained to me that if they found too much and she needed radiation, she wasn't going to accept it; she'd readied herself to die. She was in her late 80s. She came through the operation better than expected and no radiation was required but it was a slow recovery. We had to explain to Dad time and again that she was very ill and couldn't visit him. He didn't understand.

'She's whoreing around, isn't she? I know that little bitch. You wait until I see her.'

His vile words towards her were a reminder of his abuse towards me. It didn't get any better a month later when she was well enough to visit him again. Each day she'd take him in the newspaper and an iced coffee as he wasn't eating and dropping weight quickly. She tried so hard to be as attentive as she once was – anything to keep him calm.

It was a Wednesday in September after Father's Day. I took another day off work to take Mum shopping, followed by a visit to Dad. It was a cold morning and I pulled up to their house and made my way into the kitchen. Mum had her shopping list ready and instructed me on what errands we were to run first.

'OK, Jack, I've got to visit your father but let's put him fifth on the list. I need to get a few other things done before I face the verbal onslaught.'

She had a lot to take in of late. She was weak from her illness and he was speaking to her with a raised voice about her 'running around the streets at night with other men'.

The phone rang and I picked it up.

'Hello, Ellwood' residence. Jackie speaking.'

'Put Mum on.' It was Anne. Her voice was quivering. I knew immediately Dad was dead.

'Mum, come here and sit down. It's Anne.'

I helped her to her seat and handed her the phone, holding her wrinkled hand with the other. Anne spoke and Mum grabbed her chest in horror. Her head dropped.

Dad had passed away in his sleep during the early hours. Staff went in to wake him that morning and he was gone. In retrospect, we felt it was timely because he was getting worse. We knew of other parents who'd dwindled in no man's land for years on end and we didn't want that for him. When I eventually spoke with Anne, I asked to visit him. I had to say goodbye in my own way, but I didn't cry. I waited until most of the family were together, and then made my way to the aged care home. I was guided into his room by a nurse and told that I could take as much time as I wanted.

'Your dad was a lovely man; he was a joy to everyone he met,' she said.

There it was. Even in death, people who were complete strangers were telling me what a wonderful bloke he was. If he was good to others, that's nice for them. But he wasn't really good, was he?

My father's words rang in my ears: 'Never speak ill of the dead.'

'Yes, he was. Thank you very much.' I smiled and nodded.

If being a parent were a job, and you had to interview for the role, how many people would be turned away at the application process? Exactly. It would be millions per year. Saying lots and lots would be my normal mathematical rule of thumb. I'm not saying my dad was the worst of applicants but he truly wasn't right for the role. Someone should have told him, 'I'm sorry, but on further review we aren't going to take your application of being a good parent and husband any further as we feel it's not a career you would gain great satisfaction from. Maybe consider applying for a role as a publican. Have you ever thought of owning your own pub? It's a lifestyle of being around a lot of alcohol and women and if you support the local community cricket and footy club sponsorship, everyone will see you as a good bloke.' He would have aced it for sure. His grandfather had.

I took a seat next to his body. He was wearing his RM Williams chinos and plaid shirt. A pale blue cotton waffle blanket covered part of his legs too, as though they didn't want him to get too cold. The staff had also placed a late blooming daffodil from the garden in his hands that were resting on his chest. His skin was yellowing and looked paper-thin. His face was hollowing. His body now spiritless.

I didn't know what I was going to say but I knew this was my last chance to say anything. I felt cowardly because I couldn't muster up the confidence previously. I felt like a fool about to speak to a body without him actually in it but I tried. I heard Jason's voice. *Just relax.*

'Hey, Dad. I hope you weren't in pain when you passed over. I hope it was as peaceful as they say it is.'

I'd read it in books, the white light and all. I was drawing a blank. I wanted to thank him for the positives he allowed me to experience, such as private school and travel when I was younger, but being a good provider doesn't make a good parent. Living in a big beautiful home with a swimming pool and tennis court and being driven places in European cars doesn't bring you love and safety.

I placed my hand on top of his and it was frigid. I hoped it would inspire conversation even if it were one-sided, but nothing came, so I just sat. I was embarrassed that I felt as though I was wasting time. For the life of me, I just couldn't bring myself to see his loss as a reason to grieve. It was almost a relief; my siblings waiting their turn at home would have been horrified.

Then I didn't try to say anything. I just spoke my mind.

'I don't think I'm going to grieve your passing. There's no reason to. I'll be there for Mum as she's going to need support. I know you'll be happy about that. I'll go home now and fill the house with flowers from the garden just as you liked.'

I continued. 'I want you to know I stole from you when I was young. It's no excuse, but the reason I did it was because you took from me each time you abused me. I wanted you to pay and you did, you just didn't know it. You never missed it as there was so much.'

I briefly laughed. 'If I'd have been clever, I should have saved it up and run away from you but how does a kid run away towards something they don't know will better to where they're running from? I didn't have it in me to be street smart like you. So, I spent it mainly on friends. It made other people happy. You always said being charitable was important, so I was.'

Now I felt as though I really was taking up valuable time. Anne was next in line; she wanted time with him. I rose and kissed his forehead; again, so cold.

'I've always loved you. See you later.'

I've always hated saying goodbye, even in these circumstances.

It was my job to sort through old photos for the PowerPoint montage to be played at the funeral. That afternoon, while sorting, I expressed frustration at the process. 'This is complete bullshit.'

Anne and Jane were stunned at my words.

'I am going through literally hundreds of photos and there are maybe twelve of Mum, all with Dad.'

'So? That's good. You're looking for images of him for his funeral.'

I was so resentful. 'You don't get it do you, Jane? He was in everything; our life revolved around him. Where are the family pictures? Or, better still, where are the pictures of Mum? Don't answer that, I can tell you. She was behind the fucking camera taking the shots because he had to be front and centre of everything. George in the front of the house "he built". George at his business. George receiving a community award. George overseas on business for his charity work. George holding a certificate of recognition being nominated for Australian of the Year Local Hero. He was a prick and yet he had to shine.'

Mum had entered the room upon hearing my noise. I hung my head, feeling the weight, resigned to the fact that I was going to grieve the next few weeks out of anger for unresolved issues, not because I was going to miss him. Call it what you want – daddy issues – it just was.

Jane spoke up, always seeing the positive side. 'It's OK, Jack. We all knew he was like that. But look, you have your trip to Bali coming up and you really need a break. When is it again?'

I took another deep breath. 'I'm meant to be leaving in five days and he's going to fuck that up for me too. Sorry, I didn't mean to say that.'

'Oh, crap.' Jane looked stunned.

Mum chimed in. 'I'm calling the funeral home; I've got an idea.'

He'd only been dead for maybe twelve hours, but Mum was now on a mission. She knew immediately what we all wanted and that was to have a private funeral just for the immediate family first. He had always surrounded himself with yes people and we didn't want their company. So we closed ranks.

After we all said our goodbyes to him on the Saturday, I had Angus organised to be looked after by family friends and I was off to Bali by Monday – a country I'd never visited. I fell in love with it all. The kindness of the people, their religious practices, the crazy traffic, the undulating peaks and surrounding forests and the peace it brought me. I spent the following ten days in paradise getting over a difficult few months. I had time to write a eulogy for the next service, a public service for those who knew Dad as a friend through his sporting endeavours as a young man, business and his charity work. All four of us were to speak about Dad and our memories; my difficulty was I had to reflect on the small positives I could find. I found meditation brought about a different perspective, a clearer vision that I was to write about.

The day after I returned from Bali was the second service. He'd been such a pillar of his local community and Mum knew a lot of people wanted to pay their respects. As the day arrived, the sun shone and they walked into the reception centre with a lone bagpiper playing a haunting rendition of Amazing Grace, his favourite tune. The day was a success as far as wake services go. I shook so many hands of people who told me over and again what a great man my father was and how proud he would have been of all his children.

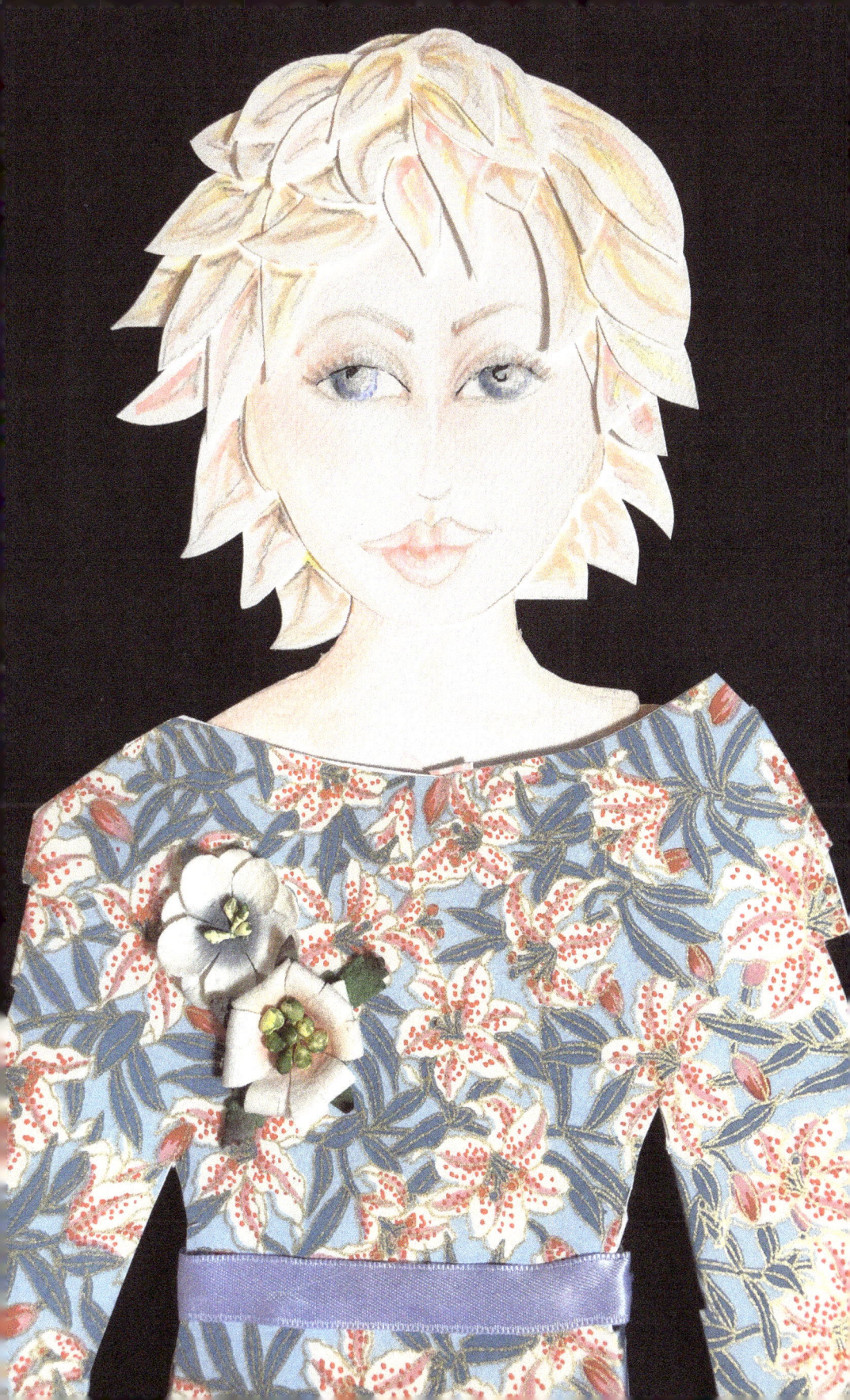

Funnily enough, Jane and I had a running joke on the day. She was waiting for someone to turn up introducing themselves as Dad's love child from one of the affairs he'd had over time.

Mum insisted I took my trip with Jason to Bali, rushing Dad's cremation through, because thirty years prior Mum's best friend had lost her son in a tragic workplace accident. Sebb was like a cousin to me and he'd died when he was felling trees in a Gippsland forest. As the tree he cut was falling to the ground, a large branch fractured and was flung into the air. It pierced his chest and killed him instantly. He was only twenty-six. At the time Mum told Dad that they had to change their holiday plans immediately to get up to Traralgon in country Victoria to help the family and attend the funeral. Dads' response was typical.

'For fuck's sake, Elizabeth, I'm not changing my plans for a big thumping upstart like him. I never liked him and he's not stuffing up my holiday.'

I'd never forgotten it, nor had Mum and, finally, she was having the last say.

When my father died, my mother blossomed. It was the most beautiful thing to witness.

2017

It only took a few months for David to contact me again, wanting to have access to Angus in the form of a few hours each Sunday. He sent Angus an email telling him he would no longer make contact with him unless Angus contacted him directly, without either mine or Jason's knowledge. What David didn't understand was that Angus and I have a very close bond – he wouldn't go behind my back.

How do you speak with a person who'd rejected their own child and taken no responsibility? I couldn't. I was no longer angry. I was exhausted. I asked Jason to take my role as head communicator; I had reached my limit. I knew I could either still play my part and be ignored or Jason could step in, knowing full well David would become even more pissed off. To come up against another man was beyond insulting to him.

In a culmination of flurried text messages, exchanged between Jason and David, a final wedge was driven into David's and my already battered relationship. We needed David to understand that Angus became distressed and anxious when he questioned why he wasn't contacting him directly, surpassing Jason and I. It was then David saw fit to hurtle abuse towards both of us with everything he could muster to make us look like the bad guys. I was merely grateful that it was all written down in case any legal action needed to be taken. He sent the words of a man who had lost his grip on his child. He had chosen his new wife over his son and no amount of desperate crawling to catch his grip on the top of the pile was going to work. And it was then he lost his footing in the eyes of a little boy.

Needing to move forward, I was back seeing Sophie to process David's behaviour again. Even family and friends tried to help me make sense of David's behaviour for what seemed like forever. I could at last breathe without thinking about repercussions if I made the wrong move. But I finally knew I wasn't the one making the wrong move.

It was around this time I made the decision to sell my home next to Jane. This time it was for positive reasons, unlike the past where I'd always been reactive, not proactive.

I'd heard of a new secondary school that I thought Angus would benefit from greatly. Darcy was getting ready to go to university. Moving meant we'd all be much closer in proximity and then eventually live together as a family. It was perfect timing that, once we unpacked into our new home and settled, I received a call from my media advisor from Women's Health East. They let me know that there was a local government program called Opening Doors and I was asked to interview for it, eventually being accepted into the 2018 class.

Opening Doors was a volunteer community program that supported candidates in making their local community more socially inclusive. I developed leadership skills and learned to understand how I could personally contribute meaningfully within my community. It was during my time there that I had a vision of combining my passion for both art and my role as a media advocate into a project I named Whesper Doll.

My career in visual merchandising taught me about the making of dolls and mannequins, as well as their role within society and how they represented women as whole. My hope was that Whesper would assist in starting discussions regarding domestic violence, sexual assault and mental health issues. My original Whesper doll was a 64-centimetre, handmade paper doll. Her name originated from the first three letters of Women's Health East, where I was a part of the Speaking Out program.

Speaking Out was a program designed to ensure that the voices of women who have experienced family violence and sexual assault were heard through the media and public events.

Her name was a play on the word 'whisper', a reflection on when women felt they couldn't speak or express themselves due to the trauma they experienced. I had firsthand experience of this and then later listened to other past victims of domestic or sexual abuse. I understood that we can have such trouble speaking, even in therapy as I'd encountered, because we are ashamed or embarrassed about our experiences.

During therapy I felt enormous physical pain in my throat when it was my time to speak and I was unable to get the words out, which resulted in my abuser mocking me and calling me crazy and delusional.

My goal and purpose is to help women within my community make a Whesper doll, an image of themselves. I do this by assisting and advocating for art therapists.

To me, it was through the process of drawing on paper or card, then cutting and sanding a version of myself, then colouring it with different mediums including pencil that I could still visualise in my mind what my abusers left behind in their wake. I was then able to dress my doll in paper clothes, which signified covering my truth, revealing it only when I felt safe and seeing it for what it truly was. It's through reflecting on what I have experienced that I can look back and see that to society a doll, which is in most forms a picture of 'perfection', doesn't depict the truth. It's an illusion we've been sold; it's nothing of what a child, let alone a real woman, should be.

I now know I deserve to be accepted, without question, for what I am: a woman with a serious mental illness, one with so many faults that I'm OK with now. I have lost the company of so many people in my life because they felt uncomfortable just knowing I had bipolar – they just couldn't accept it. They were fearful I didn't fall into what is seen as 'normal'. I no longer wish to be charming, graceful and witty for someone else because that's 'how it's meant to be' and how I was raised.

I reached a point a few years back where I wanted to lay bare the marks of years of abuse to myself, by myself and others. When I sat still and reflected on what I'd been through I grieved like never before. I finally saw the truth that wasn't masked by keeping busy, broad smiles and sweet-voiced, never-ending apologies. I saw that in the past I had continually tried to justify my shortcomings, which were ultimately just illusions played out in my mind to keep me in my place. That was on me, no one else.

The last challenge I've had to finally overcome is when life goes terribly wrong, I now get out of bed, get dressed and face it. It's the external events of women and children losing their lives to fathers, brothers, husbands and boyfriends, though, that leave me reeling the most. I try to justify continually in my head why, at times, there is no justice. I'm learning that I'm worth more being a part of the conversation to eradicate what is bleeding into our society. I don't want to give up anymore, especially on those who no longer have a voice.

From the earliest I can remember, I just wanted grow up in a loving home, with parents who I felt supported me in growing up into a strong and independent woman rather than one who was so often lost. I wanted more than anything to live a life that wasn't inflicted by twenty-four hours of non-stop grief until I tried to give up. Mine is a story about a woman living with bipolar who didn't have a choice when it came to seeing things clearly, but I'm proud of the woman I have become so far. I'm proud that no matter what life was like before, I got through it. I'm lucky that when I felt I couldn't cope, I didn't stop trying to get up. I'm glad that I kept attempting life the best I could when others felt I should have stayed down where, in their eyes, I belonged. I'm blessed that when I tried to permanently check out things didn't go to plan, that I had one parent who knew what was wrong and right eventually.

I can't reverse time, though, as much as I wanted to so I could have had my time again. I had to harness what it was I went through, as shocking to me as it was, and use my experience to help others in need. Eventually, even in a small way, I hope I can help.

I choose to no longer look at my life as what could have been if I were a stronger person, but instead I see myself as a stronger person than I've ever been. Each day I feel gratitude for what my life was, even after the abuse. Now I can reflect and gain a greater perspective, which allows me peace.

2021

As much as we all despise lockdown, it is a necessity now, but it's no longer as intriguing as I first thought. There was a moment of normality that I took for granted and then it was gone, replaced with new routine that came without a handbook. Once, a visit to our local supermarket was an ordinary chore and next it became a rare outing I looked forward to. It wasn't unusual to witness arguments about rationing toilet paper, pasta and rice. The Sunday afternoon the government announced the first lockdown in Victoria, I witnessed customers stripping packets of seeds from shelves in a local nursery. In their minds, we had reached the final apocalypse. Well, we hadn't but their fear was palpable. Scanning in via a bar code and wearing masks became the new black. Our family's blessing, though, is that we live in a country that's basically a bloody huge island.

Angus is now heading into his final years of high school and I would like to write that he never mentions David, but it's not the case. He says he's found purpose in those who love him but his biological father still stands in his periphery as a reminder of what Angus perceives as being his own fault.

As if adolescence on top of COVID isn't difficult enough, at times general light conversation can lead to him baring his thoughts regarding fears that if David were to make contact he wouldn't be strong enough to rebuke his advances. By nature Angus is a sensitive person and can become quite philosophical which often doesn't often allow him to let major issues glide by. He feels he needs to unravel and then dissect events, unfortunately leading to anger at himself, pivoting to low self-esteem and then bouts of depression.

'I know if Dad made contact, he'd be so nice that I'd forgive anything he'd done and I would allow him back into my life, but I also know in my heart if it were to happen, he'd leave and I'd be left wondering what I'd done wrong again. It just plays in my mind constantly, like I'm obsessed with it. I just want it to stop,' he says.

I'm left longing that we'll eventually get to a point where it's not a prominent issue anymore, and even though I lived through David's abuse, I was an adult. Angus was a little boy, just as I was with my father. My life experiences are many; therefore, my perspective holds more logical outcomes that I use as a compass. The events I experienced, good and bad, leave my mind balanced while my child was merely starting out on his life's journey.

Angus unequivocally loved us both, but David's actions have left a hole no one can fill. He is seeing a paediatric psychologist to help calm his mind and give him tools to allow him to hopefully see the future in a more positive light.

To feel that yearning for a parent's love, it's overwhelmingly cruel if it isn't reciprocated. The key to staying balanced is accepting the situation for what it is without self-blame. Moving forward to live a full life – that's what Angus deserves. This doesn't mean that those thoughts of 'what if' will never return, and I have to remind Angus to be conscious of living in the now, as crap as it feels.

There will always be professional help available to access over many platforms but I have to let him know that from tried experience over the years, unless you are dealing with a serious mental illness, no one can ever step in and fix how you feel. It's no secret.

I found there was no friend or stranger, pill, drink or recreational drug, number one bestseller or faith that filed any hurt or void I experienced. If it did it was ever so brief and then the grief resurfaced stronger than before. From my own experience, unless there is a chemical imbalance that needs immediate medical intervention, I'm the only person who is going to save me. Today if I ever feel low or out of sorts I can honestly say there is an outside influence that is driving my mindset to feel unsettled therefore I need to work out how to realign my thinking.

It is through a blend of loving support, professional help, tried and tested mental health tools that can start the move towards recovery from abuse. Emotional abuse lingers much longer that the physical. I will forever stand alongside Angus on the path to becoming more resilient to outside events.

It will be a good day when he decides he will no longer take on the guilt for his father's behaviour. I'm hopeful that he'll view cutting ties with David as being the best thing he ever did, but only the future will close that chapter and I'm not in charge of his narrative.

Angus says, 'Mum I'll visit him one day when I have my drivers licence and I'll ask why he listened to Olivia and just gave up on me. I want to know if he thinks about me.'

I still feel enormous guilt over what went on but then Angus says it's not my fault. If anyone needed to protect him, ultimately, it was me. I'll always see it as I didn't do anything until it was too late.

When there are moments of being out of lockdown, we visit my mother Elizabeth every Monday after school. She is now in her 90s and can view her past life in a good and bad light as she recalls what role she played with a child who was abused, then found over years had a serious mental illness. The blame game doesn't exist but is spoken about at times with regret and sorrow. She was never maternal but adores Angus and the time they have together. That is all that matters to me.

Wednesdays after school are marked for Granny Emmie. Angus and her share such an amazing bond. Her home is somewhere he learns to cook or just to sit and pass the time, chatting about nothing in particular. David's siblings have taken Angus under their wings and embraced him, giving a strong sense of self outside of our immediate family.

Jason now stands beside me stronger than ever and I am now a part of a family I always wanted. His being there doesn't magically take away any grievances I'm experiencing but he is a sounding board and we share so much, including a ridiculous sense of humour that keeps me buoyant.

What is wonderful isn't the thought of everything being perfect but instead being in total agreement that we will never reach such a level. As for completing one another: I couldn't put that weight on anyone, even though he does have extremely broad shoulders. The love we share is immeasurable.

Ultimately, all Jason ever wants is for Angus and I to be happy. I am so grateful that he didn't give up on me when I felt that taking all the burden was the only way to rid myself of guilt for not being stronger or precise in my execution of everyday happenings. He is not only a positive influence on Angus, but a mentor, always there to show through his actions that strength of character comes from staying on course and taking responsibility for your own behaviour rather than one where instant gratification is constantly required. Jason lived through domestic abuse himself so he understands Angus' grief. He raised an amazing young woman in Darcy alongside his ex-wife. She has this absolute strong sense of self, where she never doubts her capacity to live on an even playing field, knowing internally it's just expected. Now a qualified nurse completing her Masters and grad year in mental health, Darcy is always there for Angus as his best friend and sister.

Anne and Jane left home before the serious abuse started and had no idea what had been happening under our parents' roof until I was able to verbalise it well into my forties. I'm just grateful for the love and care they showed me from the time I was a little.

My brother Alex is a wonderful father to his children and acknowledges what he went through. But he has blocked out so much and I needed to learn that we all have our own story – I am in no position to undermine his version of events. What I know for sure is that his children are so fortunate to have such a dedicated father.

My brother-in-law, Andrew, will always be the first ever positive male role model in my life. From the time I met him as a twelve-year-old, he showed incredible patience and eventually took time away from his own young family to help guide me on a path less destructive.

Clair is now halfway through studying for a degree in counselling and continues to stand by my side no matter the circumstances. When I lost my way, she put me back on track as a best friend should. She has always been straightforward, willing to listen without interruption then stand up at the end and say what it was I needed to hear, not necessarily what I wanted to hear. She's my 'sister from another mister', my rock.

Scarlett, too – her unique energy and no-nonsense approach allowed me the benefit of a different perspective, especially when I would carelessly deliberate with myself that I had everything under control therefore to go off my medication was plausible.

Most importantly, these two beautiful women were there for me to laugh with until my face was aching or cry because my heart was.

So with the love and support of the family and friends around me, I have the strength to go through everything that life has to offer. I'm no longer scared to attempt life because fear dictates my actions. I am no longer a chameleon – changing myself to suit others is an insult to the person I have grown into. We are all learning how to get through life. I am no different but I am no longer in survival mode. Instead, I breathe into challenges, knowing that I'm growing from the experiences no matter how hard.

Now when I sleep, my mind is more often calm than not; my frequent nightmares have been replaced with dreams of flying over water, viewing colourful fish swimming near the surface or sitting on the ocean floor as they swim around me.

I know now that I'm an intelligent woman and am no longer seeking permission or requesting help from others to work out how to behave or live. There are times I have to protect myself from outside events that can seep into everyday life unexpectedly and doing that no longer makes me weak – I view it as preserving my energy for more valuable lessons. My focus now is on the importance of my own family and keeping myself healthy so that life can be enjoyed by us all. I want to be the best person I can be, not only to raise my son but to show that living with bipolar isn't a defect. It's an incredible opportunity to view the world from a very contrasting perspective where there are no limitations to what I can create and for that I truly feel fortunate.

Finding an Anchor in the Midst of the Storm:
Help for Women in Abusive Relationships

By Susan Marryatt
– psychotherapist and mental health social worker

The Big Picture –
violence is never ok, and you are not alone

The Family Violence Protection Act Victoria (2008) describes family violence as: A behaviour by a person towards a family member of that person, which is physically, sexually, emotionally, psychologically or economically abusive; or is threatening or coercive, or in any other way controls or dominates the family member and causes that family member to feel fear for their own or another person's safety or wellbeing. It also covers behaviour that causes a child to hear or witness the above abusive behaviours toward family members.

In Victoria, from July 2019 to June 2020, there were 88,214 family violence incidents reported to police, up 5,563 incidents from the previous year. Of these, 90% of cases occurred in the home, with children being present in 29.8% of incidents. In 48.8% of these cases, criminal charges were laid and 14.8% cases resulted in family violence notices or intervention orders (Police Crime Statistics 2019/20).

The perpetrator in 80% of family violence (FV) cases reported to Police is a male family member, and the victims, women and children. Family Violence is a huge health and safety cost to our Victorian community. According to a 2004 Vic Health Report, family violence contributes to 8% of the total disease burden for women in Victoria aged 15-44, and is the leading preventable contributor to death, disability and illness in these women. The two most common illnesses mentioned in the report were anxiety and depression (Vic Health, 2004). Family violence exceeded smoking, alcohol use, body weight and high blood pressure as the highest risk factor contributing to illness in this age group of women.

Family violence exists in our homes, schools and workplaces and impacts one in five Victorian women at some point in their adult life (VIC Health, 2010). You or a woman you care about will have been affected.

I want to acknowledge here that men are victims of violence also, and sometimes the abuser is their female partner. This does occur and these men are strongly encouraged to seek support (see support service listing at the end of this chapter). Likewise, family violence can occur within same sex relationships and family violence services are developing better responsiveness to clients who identify as LGBTIQ+. However, Police and ABS statistics (ABS 2017) show us that men are more likely to be abused by an unrelated male, and that in reported family violence, the majority of perpetrators are a male family member, with women and children most commonly being the victims.

The Australian Bureau of Statistics Personal Safety Survey (ABS 2017) found that of the women who had experienced family violence and had children in their care, 59% reported that children had witnessed the violence. In addition, according to 2016 Australian crime statistics, children are present in one-third of family violence cases reported to police.

Many women I have worked with over the years come to counselling with the questions: Why did it happen to me? Why does he treat me this way? These are complex questions to answer, and many factors can contribute to why a man chooses to use violence to control his partner:

- He makes a choice to use violence.
- Misogyny and male sense of privilege over women.
- A broader community acceptance of violence.
- Childhood abuse and family modelling of using abusive behaviour for controlling others.

Sometimes there are red flags early in the relationship, that a new partner may be controlling or abusive, sometimes there are not. In any case, his angry behaviour may be explained away or forgiven. Most women I have talked with reported a pattern of abuse that built up slowly over time and worsened when life was stressful or when children came into the family. Walsh (2008) found that 20% of pregnant Australian women surveyed, reported experiencing physical or emotional abuse by their partner, with 6% stating that physical violence had increased during pregnancy. Nearly all the women I have worked with said that they hoped things would change over time and he would become less abusive.

Some tried to stand up to their partner's abuse, often with harsh consequences.

Women are often ready to seek help when a bottom line has been crossed. For some this might be a physical or sexual assault, for others it can be cutting her off from family and friends, or cruelty to children or pets. Sometimes a close friend or relative notices that she is struggling. In any case, women can be assured that there are confidential, caring and professional services available to help them whether they are thinking of leaving the relationship or staying. Counsellors and social workers at family violence services are usually female, they will believe you, and will work with you to increase your safety and wellbeing, and that of your children. I encourage any woman reading this who is unsure about her safety in her relationship, to take that first step.

A woman's experiences in childhood can make her vulnerable to tolerating abusive behaviour, and less likely to seek support outside of the relationship. I want to be very clear that no woman (or child) asks to be abused or controlled, however sometimes because of her own history or current circumstances it may be very difficult for a woman to leave the relationship, or she may be vulnerable to further abusive relationships.

I want to illustrate this further with a concept called the Shark Cage®. I first encountered this concept some years ago at a family violence forum where it was introduced by workers from a women's family violence program. It was developed by Melbourne psychologist Ursula Benstead, who has used the framework to educate and empower women who have been in abusive relationships to 'renovate' their own shark cage of human rights and increase their capacity to move away from people who use abusive behaviours. This reduces the risk of becoming entangled in long-term relationships with abusive men (Benstead, 2021).

The 5-Step Shark Cage Framework (Ursula Benstead, 2018)

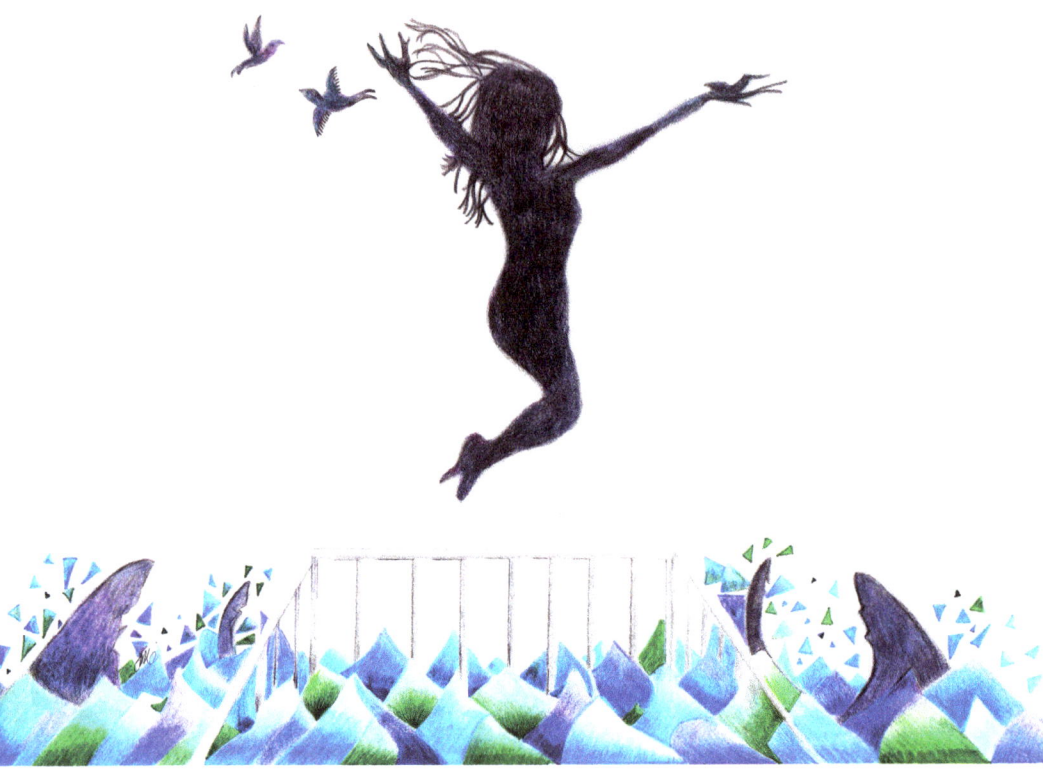

1. The Shark Cage Metaphor.

The shark cage represents our boundaries that help us to maintain physical, psychological and emotional safety from anyone who aims to exploit or abuse us. We aren't born with a shark cage; it is up our families in childhood, schools and media to help us develop a sense of our rights, which builds the foundations of our first shark cage (Benstead, 2020).

The bars of the shark cage represent a right that each woman has: I have the right to be treated with respect; I have the right to say no; I have the right to choose how I spend my time. If we have a supportive and nurturing childhood, where adults protect and respect children, we learn that we possess these rights and develop the skills required to maintain them or take a stand if our rights are dismissed. Our shark cage of human rights is not designed to keep us separated from others. Having a sense of our boundaries and rights enhances our capacity for recognising and maintaining healthy and mutually respectful relationships (Benstead 2021).

Often when women have experienced emotional, physical or sexual abuse during childhood, the bars of our shark cage have not been strongly installed, some may be missing. Likewise, women who have been in abusive partnerships have had their bars (or boundaries) damaged and have a different experience of safety to women with a wellbuilt shark cage. Jackie refers to her childhood experiences of emotional and physical abuse, as well as a sexual assault at age 19, to which her mother responded with little concern for her wellbeing. These experiences left Jackie with a belief that abusive behaviour was a normal part of sex and close relationships. This in turn left her vulnerable to further abuse by future partners.

2. Renovating the Shark Cage

Healing and recovering from abuse means renovating our shark cage. A woman can recognise ways that she may be at risk to abusive men by exploring this in counselling, group therapy or by self-education.

What bars are missing from her shark cage that need to be installed? How has she been misled or exploited in the past? What does safety and wellbeing mean to her? What does a healthy, respectful relationship look like? What new skills may need to be developed for the woman to take a stand for her rights when it is safe to do so? Benstead (2021) explains that once the bars are in place, sharks bang up against them and may find it harder to hurt women and have opportunities for further contact.

3. Installing the Alarm System

Every shark cage needs an alarm system that alerts the woman that her rights have been breached and a boundary crossed. One of the most efficient systems is our intuition and bodily feeling. Something is not right here for me. I don't feel safe or I don't like the way this man is looking at me. My stomach is churning, and my jaw is tense – that means I'm feeling anxious! There has been a boundary violation and I need to say something or get away from him.

The alarm might be raised by something he says: 'This guy is constantly running down his ex-wife, he's not taking responsibility for his part in his marriage breakdown. His language about her is disrespectful'.

Benstead (2018) outlined her process in group work with women to ask them to think of a recent incident where they may have had a boundary crossed and explore which right had been threatened, how they responded. With the group, she explored what assertive actions could be tried, whilst prioritising safety always. Benstead referred to encouraging her clients to practise tuning into their bodily signals three times during their day, so that their internal alarm system becomes fine-tuned and connected rather than disconnected.

4. *Learning How to Defend Potential Breaches of the Shark Cage*
This part of the process is about assertiveness training. For women who have experienced control and abuse from a young age they may not know how to assert their rights and may confuse aggression with assertiveness. Benstead (2011) explains that sometimes it's a case of fake it until we make it: if we expect that others treat us with respect, and we treat ourselves with respect, we will eventually find that we do respect and value ourselves.

In counselling and women's group work, we examine the behaviours of the assertive woman: how does she stand, use eye contact and tone of voice to make her message clear, without putting herself at greater risk? We give the women homework assignments to practise assertiveness, e.g., saying no to the neighbour who drops in without phoning or her brother who often calls asking to borrow money. Women often worry that they will be considered a bad or selfish person if they don't say yes and please others. This idea needs to be explored in terms of what is reasonable and that selfcare is not being selfish.

This learning of assertive behaviour can take some practise and requires good coaching. However once women learn the skills and put them into practise, they begin to see and feel the benefits for their wellbeing and selfconfidence and the flow on benefits for their children and family members.

5. *Identifying the Early Warning Signs of Potential Sharks*

The following checklist, Look Before You Leap, is a useful resource for women to read and discuss with their friends, sisters and daughters. I compiled the checklist in 2009 when I was providing women's family violence support groups at a community health centre. The various characteristics of men who are abusive were listed by women in the groups as well as from family violence literature, and reflected common experiences of women early in their relationships with previous partners.

Sometimes women attending counselling become aware through working with the Shark Cage framework that their current partner is controlling and abusive. It becomes a difficult process to really face up to what this means in terms of living within the partner's cycle of abuse, with periods of calm, even loving times followed by a buildup of tension to reoccurrences of jealous, controlling and abusive behaviour. As women speak up more, tension increases in the relationship and abuse can become more frequent and more severe.

As counsellors, we advise women that there are only two ways that the violence can stop in their relationship:

1. The abuser takes responsibility for his abusive behaviour by getting professional help to change (such as a men's behaviour change program).

2. The woman leaves the relationship and may require legal protection, such as an intervention order, as well as a carefully planned safety exit plan.

The Shark Cage framework is useful in helping women to answer that question of why do I attract these men who want to control and abuse me? Women can see where elements that uphold their human rights may be missing from their shark cage and where the alarm system has been damaged or disconnected by experiences of abuse early in life. The Shark Cage can be strengthened by supportive, professional counselling or women's family violence group programs. Exploring this framework can help women to understand patterns of abuse in their lives and give them a sense of agency to change these patterns. It is important to emphasise that having a strong shark cage of rights will be immensely helpful to a woman, but it cannot provide a guarantee against further abuse. Only abusive men can control and are responsible for their abusive behaviour. In addition, the picture of why family violence occurs is much bigger than an individual woman and her experiences.

Family violence occurs first and foremost because of community attitudes that allow violence against women to prevail, attitudes of disrespect and sexism, together with minimisation of women's right to be safe. The fact that some men still choose to control their partners through intimidation and abusive behaviours is evidence that these broader societal attitudes exist.

In her recent memoir, The Fictional Woman, Tara Moss (2014) gives us an excellent manifesto of the ways in which women are stereotyped and often reduced by labels and attitudes to Madonna or whore status. This mythology contributes to girl's and women's reports of sexual assault being minimised or disputed by the people that should believe and protect them. Women can educate themselves on the stats and facts around family violence in Australia and read victim survivors stories on excellent websites such as ANROWS and Our Watch (2022) www.ourwatch.org.au. There is a service directory in the next section listing Victorian and national support services.

I deeply thank Jackie for having the courage, compassion and determination to write her story in this memoir. I'm sure it will encourage girls and women who read it to speak up when they feel unsafe and to access the support that will increase their safety and their options.

There is help for you and someone will listen.

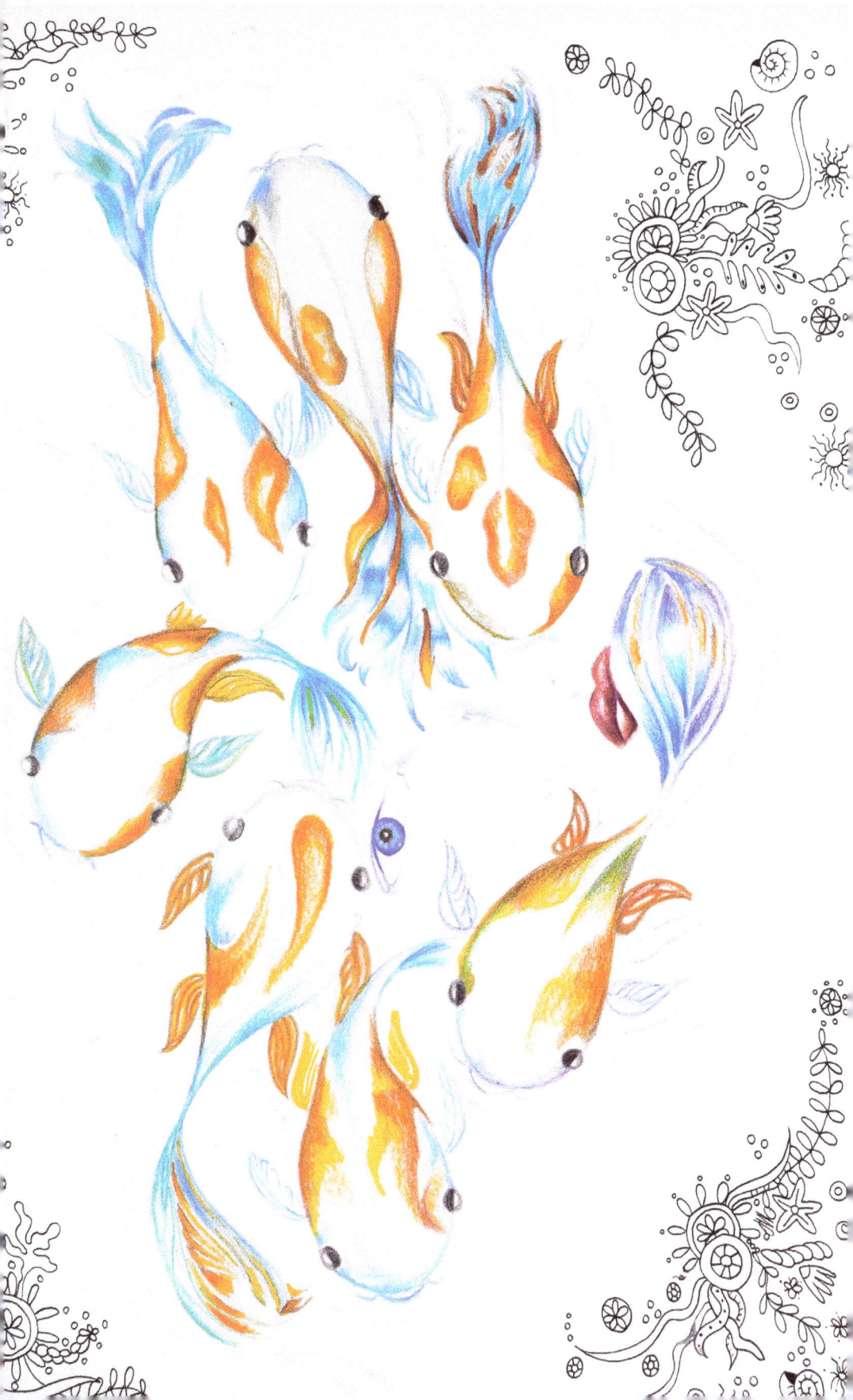

References

Australian Bureau of Statistics 2016, *Personal Safety Survey*, Australian Bureau of Statistics.

Benstead, U 2011, 'The Shark Cage: The use of metaphor with women who have experienced abuse', *Psychotherapy in Australia*, vol. 7, no. 2.

Benstead, U 2018, *The Shark Cage® Group Program Manual: A Human Rights Approach to Empowerment & Healing for Women Who Have Experienced Sexual Assault or Family Violence*, Psychology Press, Australia.

Benstead, U 2020, The Shark Cage Metaphor Animation, www.thesharkcage.com.

Benstead, U 2021, *The Shark Cage Framework: How to Spot A Shark: A Five Step Guide to Avoiding Relationships with Controlling and Abusive Men*.

McKenzie, M 2012, 'Strengthening the Shark Cage', *DVRC Quarterly*, ed. 3, spring/summer.

Moss, T 2014, *The Fictional Woman*, Harper Collins, Australia.

Our Watch website (2022) www.ourwatch.org.au

Victorian Health Promotion Foundation 2004, *The Health Costs of Violence: Measuring the Burden of Disease Caused by Intimate Partner Violence. A Summary of Findings*, Victorian Health Promotion Foundation, Melbourne.

Walsh, D 2008, 'The hidden experience of violence during pregnancy: a study of 400 pregnant Australian women', *Australian Journal of Primary Health*, vol. 14, no. 1, pp. 97-105.

Appendix A

Relationship Warning Signs:
Look Before You Leap!

When you meet a new potential partner have your antenna up for the following attitudes and behaviours that may be indicators for that person to become abusive over time.
In the first few weeks, does s/he:

- Drink too much and become aggressive when drunk?

- Become overly attentive (10 calls+ per day) so you feel like you have no space?

- Talk about moving in together or future plans – 'We were meant to be together' – when you aren't ready for this level of commitment?

- Criticise or degrade former partners/wife?

- Talk as a victim?

- Often ask you for money?

- Give you advice about your life?

- Start to tell you your friends are no good/avoid socialising with them?

- Have friends who are disrespectful to women, do drugs or crime?

- Talk disrespectfully about his mother, sisters or women in general?

In the first few months, does s/he:

- Move in even when you say/feel it's too soon?

- Start to reorganise your home?

- Start to parent your children? (The role of caring adult is more appropriate whilst they/their builds a relationship with your children.)

- Start to criticise or belittle things you do?

- Fly into sudden, irrational tempers and then downplay this behaviour?

- Use (even mild) physical control on you or your children?

- Have a fascination with violent movies, games or weapons?

- Have a history of violence toward others, intervention order, etc.?

- Have difficulty expressing his feelings?

- Mainly focus on his own needs, or compete with the children for your attention?

- Show cruelty to animals or the children?

- Demonstrate irresponsible behaviour with money or disappear for long periods, etc.?

- Pressure you into having sex when you don't want to?

- Avoid taking responsibility for his behaviour by denying it or blaming others?

- Constantly check your movements, who you are seeing, etc.?

- Control the finances, without consulting you on money decisions?

- Demand increasing amounts of your time, energy, attention or affection?

Stand back and ask yourself: what is really happening here? Talk to someone you trust about your partner's behaviour – is this respectful, healthy behaviour? Do I feel safe?

Compiled by Susan Marryatt, together with victim survivors who participated in women's FV education and support groups, 2008-2013.

Appendix B

Family Violence Services for Victim Survivors

If you or your children are in immediate risk of harm, call 000 and ask for police who have authority to intervene and protect you and your family.

Victoria

There are multiple FV services in every region of Victoria that provide counselling support and outreach/advocacy; referrals to emergency accommodation and housing, legal and financial support; parenting support and children's programs. There are specialised programs for Aboriginal and CALD people, LGBTIQ people, older persons and people with disabilities.

See the Domestic Violence Resource Centre website for services in your area: https://www.dvrcv.org.au/support-services/victorian-services

Sexual Assault Crisis Line (after hours 5pm-9am weekdays, 24 hours on weekends): 1800 806 292

Centres Against Sexual Assault (fifteen locations around Victoria). See Casa Forum website: https://casa.org.au/contact-us/

There are separate services for men who are perpetrators of family violence. If a perpetrator is seeking help, they can contact:

Men's Referral Service: 1300 766 491

No to Violence: https://ntv.org.au/

National

1800 Respect (national 24/7 sexual assault and domestic family violence counselling service): 1800 737 732

Mental Health Support

- Beyond Blue

- Lifeline

- Head to Health (post-COVID initiative of mental health intake teams to link people to local services). See website for multiple locations. **https://headtohelp.org.au**

- Bipolar Australia

- Talk to your GP about a mental health plan to see a psychologist/counsellor

- Community health services offer free counselling for mental health issues

Thank you

To Jason for your support to not only write this book but more importantly to actually finish it. I finally got there. For being a wonderful father to Darcy and Angus – you're the best of the best and then some.

To Blaise van Hecke and Kev Howlett from Busybird Publishing for giving me the confidence to actually publish and for all your hard work behind the scenes.

My editor, the incredible Anna Bilbrough. Your patience, guidance and input was wonderful even when I was at a loss to write; it was such a pleasure working with you.

Susan Marryatt, you have been an inspiration to me for over a decade. You helped me look at life in a totally different way, a healthier way, and I can never thank you enough. Now it's your turn to publish.

To Kate Ravenscroft, Kate Gibson and Ari Milecki from Women's Health East for your unwavering support from the very beginning and over the journey.

To the incredible team of women from EDVOS.

To Angus, for telling me I'm the best mum in the universe even when I don't feel like it. To Darcy, for telling me my past doesn't make me the person I am now; it actually has made me a better person for the experience of it all.

Anne and Jane, you are the best sisters I could have ever asked for. I can't thank you enough. You have always been there to love me unconditionally.

To Clair, for nearly forty years we have always spoken the same language and laughed at the most ridiculous things. When we were apart, I missed you terribly. I love you.

Scarlet, you have always been so supportive but still the voice of reason, even when I felt I was fine off my medication. Thank you for being there through the good times and bad. Your support has always meant the word to me.

Leeanne, you are no longer here but always in my heart.

Mum, I don't think you'll ever read this book because you lived through it with me and I know it exhausted you. Thank you for growing after Dad passed and thank you too for finally listening to me once the dust settled.

Thanks to Sharon Mo from Hachette Publishing for allowing me to quote from Too Soon Old, Too Late Smart by Gordon Livingston. It meant the world to me and I felt very honoured.

For more information visit:
www.twopolarbears.com.au

www.ingramcontent.com/pod-product-compliance
Lightning Source LLC
Chambersburg PA
CBHW040414100526
44588CB00022B/2827